Essential Oils
For Beginners

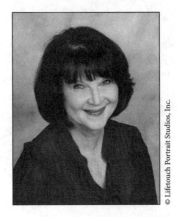

© Lifetouch Portrait Studios, Inc.

About the Author

Kac Young has been a producer, writer, and director in the Hollywood television industry for over twenty-five years. Kac has also earned a PhD in Natural Health and a Doctorate in Naturopathy. Clients come to her for advice on health, nutrition, and spiritual well-being. Using her third Doctorate degree in Clinical Hypnotherapy, she helps people with weight control, smoking cessation, behavior modification, stress reduction, past-life regression, and phobia management. She has a monthly podcast on the Surn Spiritual Network called The Art of Healing (sponsored by The Elysium Project).

Kac Young is also a licensed Religious Science Minister, a Certified Archetypal Therapist and Counselor, a Certified Meditation Teacher, a Master Feng Shui Practitioner, a Career Coach for aspiring actors and directors, and a former pilot of private airplanes. She is currently working on a black belt in Aikido and is a certified Medical Qigong instructor. She teaches classes in Crystal Healing, Essential Oils, Feng Shui, Meditation, Pendulum therapy, and Qigong.

She is active on behalf of animal rights and fostering and preserving women's rights.

Essential Oils

For Beginners

A Guide to What They Are & How to Use Them

Kac Young, PhD

Llewellyn Publications
Woodbury, Minnesota

FIRST EDITION
Second Printing, 2020

Cover design: Shannon McKuhen
Interior art: Llewellyn Art Department

Llewellyn Publications is a registered trademark of Llewellyn Worldwide Ltd.

Library of Congress Cataloging-in-Publication Data

Names: Young, Kac, author.
Title: Essential oils for beginners : a guide to what they are & how to use
  them / Kac Young.
Description: First edition. | Woodbury, Minnesota : Llewellyn Publications,
  [2020] | Includes bibliographical references and index.
Identifiers: LCCN 2019044773 (print) | LCCN 2019044774 (ebook) | ISBN
  9780738762739 (paperback) | ISBN 9780738762951 (ebook)
Subjects: LCSH: Essences and essential oils—Therapeutic use. |
  Aromatherapy.
Classification: LCC RM666.A68 Y675 2020 (print) | LCC RM666.A68 (ebook) |
  DDC 615.3/219—dc23
LC record available at https://lccn.loc.gov/2019044773
LC ebook record available at https://lccn.loc.gov/2019044774

Llewellyn Worldwide Ltd. does not participate in, endorse, or have any authority
or responsibility concerning private business transactions between our authors and
the public.

All mail addressed to the author is forwarded, but the publisher cannot, unless
specifically instructed by the author, give out an address or phone number.

Any internet references contained in this work are current at publication time,
but the publisher cannot guarantee that a specific location will continue to be
maintained. Please refer to the publisher's website for links to authors' websites
and other sources.

Llewellyn Publications
A Division of Llewellyn Worldwide Ltd.
2143 Wooddale Drive
Woodbury, MN 55125-2989
www.llewellyn.com

Printed in the United States of America

Dedication

This book is dedicated to all those curious, genius healers who have come before us and experimented with plants. Here's to the brave souls who recognized their qualities, grew them, harvested them, distilled them, and put their oils to use for the healing of humans, animals, and the planet itself.

I'm thankful for their dedication, long hours, and commitment to examine, classify, and experiment with these living species we call our friends and healers.

Oh yes, and a huge thank you to Mother Nature for thinking of all this in the first place.

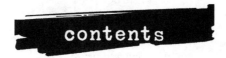

contents

Sixteen
Pine (Pinus sylvestris) Essential Oil I4I

Seventeen
Rose (Rosa × damascena) Essential Oil I47

Eighteen
Roman Chamomile (Chamaemelum nobile) Essential Oil I53

Part 3
Putting Essential Oils to Use 195

Twenty-Nine
Using Essential Oils for Mind
and Emotions 285

Thirty
Using Essential Oils for
Spirituality and Ritual 303

Final Thoughts 327

Glossary 329

Recommended Resources 333

Source Material 335

Index 339

acknowledgments

A book is a living thing. First it is the idea in the mind of the creator, then it is the work of the author, followed by editors, printers, artists, publishers, distributors, and retail sellers. Many hands go into making a book.

The first person who deserves acknowledgment is Angela Wix. She came to me with the request to write this book after working together on a previous book, *The Healing Art of Essential Oils,* and a calendar featuring essential oils. The entire Llewellyn team is a great example how teams work when creativity is inspired at the top. Thank you especially to team leader Bill Krause and editor Annie Burdick. My lovely and wonderful agent Lisa Hagan not only put the contract together for us but also had the faith in, and the support of, this project from day one. She's been incredible throughout the process. I am grateful every day for her guidance and friendship.

Michelle Stevens at The Refill Shoppe in Ventura for inviting me to speak; Katherine Dippong-Lawson for allowing me to teach my courses in aromatherapy; Aurora Heinemann for hosting me at her Yoga Channel; Rakesh Samani at Aum Shanti Bookstore, New York City, for inviting me to teach; Rev. David Bruner for asking me to come to San Jose and teach; Kelly Holland Azzaro for her input and knowledge about Animal Aromatherapy and her friendship; Kat Sanborn and Jake Kent at Llewelyn for getting me on the radio and podcasts; and all of the wonderful students who come to my classes, ask me questions, and cause me to probe further into the wonderful world of essential oils. I also want to thank the radio and podcast hosts who have had me on their shows and treated me with great respect: Dave Congalton, Dr. Paula Joyce, Gwilda Wiyaki, Monique Chapman, Servet Hasan, Hercules Invictus, Donna Seebo, Randi Fine, Brenda Michaels, Rob Spears, Pamela Atherton, Sheryl Glick, Marianne Pestana, Janeane Bernstein, Kaisha & Kelsey, Crystal Myrick, Wendy Garrett, and all the other writers and journalists who have included me in their articles, posts, and blogs. A very special thank you to Dr. Paula Joyce for encouraging me to write an A–Z guide for essential oil remedies for common human conditions. Her encouragement was the inspiration for chapter 28.

I owe the greater part of this book to all of them.

One cannot write a book without a muse, the unfathomable source of inspiration, guidance, feedback, and clandestine editorial help. For the hours of her jaunty spirit, brilliant ideas, and encouragement, I bow in gratitude for her generosity, insights, corrections, and overall unconditional love and support. Every day I am filled with gratitude for having this wonderful person at my side through thick and thin and life-altering fires, rains, and thunderstorms. Thank you, my dear Marlene Morris.

And to my wonderful friends Pamela Ventura, Lisa Tenzin-Dolma, Tracy Abbott Cook, J. Randy Taraborrelli, Jacklyn Zeman, Valerie Voss Evans, Sharon Wuerl, Donna Wells, Peggy Jones, Terry Cole-Whittaker, Hercules, Hadley Fitzgerald, and Beth Wareham all of whom continue to support me in my efforts to make a small difference in our world. Without their love and friendship, I'd be shapeless.

You give me form and inspiration. Thank you from the very bottom of my heart.

disclaimer

E ssential oils have proven historically to contain therapeutic healing properties and benefits. However, you
should not substitute the ideas and methods in this book for
traditional medical care. Seek advice from your physician
and use this book with common sense.

The information is presented for educational purposes
only and is not intended to diagnose, prescribe, prevent,
treat, mitigate, or cure medical or psychological conditions.
The information herein is not intended as medical advice but
rather a sharing of knowledge and information based on research and experience.

Each body reacts differently to natural products and essential oils, so results may vary person to person. Essential oils are potent. Use care when handling them and always do a patch test on your skin and a smell test to make sure an essential oil is compatible with your personal chemistry. Use extra caution with children and seniors. Perform your own research before using an essential oil. Always err on the side of caution.

introduction

E ssential oils seem to be in the news almost every day. I
get one or two notices a day in my inbox. Maybe you
heard about essential oils on a podcast; or you read about
them in a magazine, or a friend shared about their own use.
Whatever your personal interest in essential oils is, whether
it began as mild curiosity about the particularly beautiful
aroma of an oil you encountered in a store display, or you had
an intense experience and were intrigued with the possibilities of an oil's aroma and healing power, you are here. That's
a very good thing.

It is my pleasure to welcome you to this amazing world
of incredible natural essences that will change your life for

the better. I know it's a large claim, but in my experience, I can't recall one person who learned about essential oils who didn't benefit from having them in their life.

My enthusiasm is high; I fancy myself a goodwill ambassador for essential oils. There are so many exciting ways essential oils can enhance your life. They have physical components that can heal and aid our bodies. They are beneficial to our emotional lives. They can help us overcome feelings of sadness, grief, depression, fear, and exhaustion, and can exchange the negative feelings we experience for joy and happiness in a matter of minutes. They have spiritual components that can lift our spirits and connect us to places we never dreamed of going. If that sounds like a best friend, they are that, too. I hope I can pass along not only my enthusiasm for essential oils, but also what I have learned over the years about them and their wonderful benefits to you.

I belong to several online groups for essential oils. I am always asked, "What are your favorite essential oils, and why do you like them?" I have given my answers much thought and often reply that my first choice for an essential oil is lavender because of its various properties, aroma, and all-around appeal. For this book, I selected twenty of my top picks based on their versatility, compatibility, and helpful properties. I wanted to select twenty oils that would give you a wide variety of benefits for all areas of your life. I didn't want to neglect body, mind, or soul in this roster. You should have a balanced palette with these selected oils.

Several times a year I teach classes and give workshops in essential oils and aromatherapy. You may be familiar with my other book, *The Healing Art of Essential Oils*. That book is a culmination of thirty years working with essential oils. They have become my specialty!

Each time I begin a new class I ask the students, "What do you know about essential oils?" The answers range from "They smell good; Not much; I've used them for a few months; I just got a set for my birthday and don't know what to do with them," to "What are they, anyway?" At the end of the class or workshop I ask them, "What do you know now that you didn't know before you took this class?" Hands go up instantly, "That they are powerful; That I have to dilute them; That I should use gloves when mixing them; That there are different mixtures for different ages; You shouldn't use them on pets." It's always gratifying to know that the course was valuable, and I've sent a better-educated person out into the world of aromatherapy and essential oils.

Essential oils are perhaps the most underrated natural gifts from the earth that we can find, and they are designed especially for us. They are chemically constituted for compatibility with the human body. But you shouldn't just pick them up and start using them without some background and guidance. There is a lot to learn about essential oils and how to use them correctly, safely, and most effectively. The goal of this book is to give you the right background for a lifetime of use and enjoyment of essential oils.

When they are extracted and processed, essential oils become stronger and very potent and can be dangerous if we don't use them with care and caution. Parts of this book will instruct you on how to use essential oils properly and effectively by explaining the do's and don'ts of use. This book will also introduce you to a new world of natural products; you can make your own cleaning products, cosmetics, massage oils, aromatics, aphrodisiacs, and magical formulas.

The greatest benefits of essential oils might be in the ways they keep you green. When you use essential oils, you are choosing to help keep our planet healthy. You are choosing a sustainable product that can be renewed year after year for generations to come. You are providing jobs to growers, farmers, workers, distillers, and shippers around the world. With just one little bottle of essential oil, you become part of the legacy of caring individuals who believe planetary conservation matters. Many essential oils plants are endangered, so it is important to buy from suppliers whose products are fair market and grown as sustainable crops.

Essential oils often use fragrance to entice us before using their unique properties to heal and protect us. As members of the plant kingdom, they are meant to help themselves first and then help us; much like putting on your oxygen mask first in an airplane before helping another with theirs. Essential oils are fashioned by the plant kingdom to be compatible in many ways with the human species because we have similar biology and their unique chemistry can help us improve our lives.

The very essence of a plant's life-matter is the collection of oils and fluids that protect it from bacteria, viruses, parasites, predators, and diseases as part of the natural process of living. When extracted from the plants, these essential oils can do the same thing for humans. They are little miracle workers in a bottle.

Western medicine is a marvelous tool to diagnose what ails us. No one has perfected surgical techniques, lifesaving emergency measures, and radical transplants more than modern surgeons and specialists. The new frontier before us is to explore how essential oils can assist these wondrous measures in healing the patient without the side effects and trace evidence left behind by modern pharmaceuticals. Already, research on the effectiveness of essential oils has begun around the world. It's going to be a fantastic day when modern medicine and ancient knowledge join hands and walk together into the future of pain management and gentler natural healing.

One by one, we will explore each little miracle in dark glass bottles and learn about their properties, benefits, applications, and how we can put them to use for our health and personal empowerment.

Each essential oil has a lot of options to offer you. Some have properties that will help with congestion, some can assist you with muscle aches, and others can lift you emotionally when you're feeling down.

I'm looking forward to this journey and I hope you are too. In the first section, we'll learn the basics about essential oils to offer you a fundamental knowledge of where they came from, how they are cultivated, grown, harvested, and processed. This leads directly into an explanation of the reasons why the human body reacts to and utilizes essential oils and their extraordinary healing properties.

In chapter 1 we will journey through the ages with our essential oils and find out how ancient cultures used them and for what purpose.

Chapter 2 explains what essential oils are, what part of the plant they come from, the various means of extraction and distillation, and how they work in the human body.

Chapter 3 covers the all-important safety guidelines, and probably some interesting things you didn't know about essential oils. There are oils that are toxic and oils that should not be used by children or pregnant women. We'll discuss them all so you will feel safe using essential oils in your life. I tell you how to store and dispose of your oils for optimum care and safe handling.

In chapter 4 we will cover the practical knowledge about carrier oils, which is laid out for you along with a description of why they are vitally important, how you can use them for added benefit, and where some of them originate. Carrier oils also have hidden purposes and you'll learn about those along the journey.

Part 2 begins with chapters 5 through 24, which introduce you to the profiles of twenty essential oils: bergamot, clary sage, clove, eucalyptus, frankincense, lavender, lemon, Melissa, orange, patchouli, peppermint, pine, rose, Roman chamomile, rose geranium, rosemary, sandalwood, tea tree, thyme, and ylang-ylang. I recommend starting with these essential oils. The information you will learn in these twenty chapters will provide you with a solid basis for a long and happy life using essential oils for yourself and for your family.

Part 3 begins with chapter 25 and a wonderful introduction to blending essential oils and creating aromatic masterpieces.

Chapter 26 gives you a primer on diffusing and diffusers and how to get the best results from your airborne essential oils. I'll also give you a list of various blends you can use for different purposes.

In chapter 27 you'll find some easy recipes for face moisturizers, wrinkle creams, summer and winter applications, and some healing creams for bites, burns, and in case you find yourself entangled in some poison ivy. You'll love how simple they are to make, and you can use them not only for yourself, but as gifts for others, too.

I love chapter 28, a chapter for comprehensive remedies using essential oils. You'll find them listed A–Z for your easy access.

Chapter 29 addresses the emotional uses of essential oils. You'll find an array of choices you can use to alleviate everything from a broken heart to weight control.

In chapter 30 I share some ideas for using the sacred side of essential oils for rituals and commemorating special moments and milestones in your life and those around you. Each essential oil we discuss in this book comes with metaphysical qualities, and I've made a list of those so you can deepen your spiritual practices using essential oils.

Once again, please allow me to welcome you to the wonderful and exciting world of essential oils. They are ancient gifts from Mother Nature reemerging into our modern world. I am confident you will have a wonderful time exploring all these exciting oils and aromas.

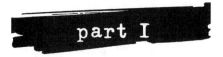

Understanding the Basics of Essential Oils

In this first section we will cover some of the fascinating history of essential oils as they made their way through the centuries into our lives. We'll discover what essential oils are, where they come from, and why they are so compatible with the human body. You'll learn some cautionary measures for using essential oils, and age-appropriate doses for applications on children, adults, and the elderly. Every essential oil needs to be diluted, so you'll learn about carrier oils and what they have to offer when paired with an essential oil. It's a fascinating look into the world of essential oils. Then, in part 2, you'll meet twenty individual essential oils up close and personal. And now, how it all began.

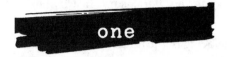

History of Essential Oils

I magine you enter a contest and win first prize. Your reward is a trip to the most luscious, exotic garden in the world. Close your eyes for a moment and imagine that you are in the middle of thousands of amazing plants and trees from around the world. There are lush, tall trees; flowering bushes; plump roses; high and low grasses; multi-colored barks; plentiful, shiny seeds; and elegant ferns in every shape and size. Some are in flower; some are dormant. As you walk around the garden, the fragrances wafting from the plants are intoxicating. You might even feel slightly light-headed because of all the perfumes competing for your attention.

One by one, you begin to identify the fragrances: some are sweet, some very floral, some hearty, earthy, spicy, pungent, sharp, and some even smell like a freshly cut Christmas tree. It's like being in the middle of nature's apothecary.

Now that you have officially entered the sumptuous world of essential oils, a place from which you will emerge changed for the better, please ask yourself a few questions: Why am I interested in essential oils? What do I want from them? What do I expect from them? Am I willing to learn how to use them wisely?

You already know in your heart if this is mild curiosity or if you are willing to shift your old ways of thinking and living in order to incorporate essential oils into your daily life. Be open. A few hours of painless study will open new avenues for you and your relationship with essential oils.

Essential oils can easily help you live a greener and more natural life, reduce toxic chemical waste in the world, and add a spiritual dimension to your life path. They can help heal you physically, emotionally, and, if you choose, spiritually.

Before we dive into the details of what oils are and how to use them, let's look at how they have been used throughout history, so we can understand them a bit better before applying them for our use.

18,000 BCE

Essential oils have been around for a very long time. They are definitely not new or the latest fad. They have longevity, character, and well-earned history.

The earliest evidence of human knowledge of the healing properties of plants was found in Lascaux, located in the Dordogne region in **France**. Cave paintings on the walls suggest the use of medicinal plants in everyday life and have been carbon dated as far back as 18,000 BCE. The excavation reports from Lascaux show the people were familiar with the properties of eight local plants and herbs, which are still used in the region today. The plants and oils were used for both cooking and healing.

4500 BCE

Evidence has shown the **Egyptians** used aromatic essential oils as early as 4500 BCE. They became renowned for their knowledge of cosmetology, ointments, and aromatic oils. In fact, Cleopatra VII went a little overboard with her use of essential oils. Legend has it that she scented the sails of her ships with essential oils as well as her garments and bed linens.

At the height of Egypt's power, priests were the only authorities allowed to use aromatic oils. It was regarded as necessary that one be united with the Gods to use them.

Egyptians were fanatical with the afterlife and wanted to insure they had material goods to survive on the other side. When King Tutankhamun's tomb was opened in 1925, 300 synoptic jars that had been previously sealed with wax 3,000 years before were found to contain a collection of sacred essential oils that still possessed the aroma of the plant they came from. The oils were designated to protect the Pharaoh as he crossed the bridge from this life to the next.

Throughout history, essential oils have been used as perfumes, as wound healers, as preservatives, for wrapping mummies, for sacred ceremonies, in consecration ceremonies, and for help with emotional and mental illnesses.

3000 BCE

The use of aromatic oils was first recorded in **China** in 3000 BCE during the reign of Huang Di, the legendary Yellow Emperor. They created balsams, perfumed oils, scented barks, resins, spices, and aromatic vinegars for everyday life. They took many of the oils and pastes from plants and transformed them into pills, powders, suppositories, medicinal cakes, and ointments. For example, in China, peppermint was used to quell nausea, to assist with childbirth, and to aid psychological illness and epilepsy.

1000 BCE

Traditional **East India** medicine called Ayurveda has a 3,000-year history of incorporating essential oils into their healing potions. Ayur means life and Veda means knowledge. Vedic literature lists more than 700 substances, including cinnamon, ginger, myrrh, and sandalwood as effective for healing and pain abatement.

During the outbreak of the bubonic plague, Ayurveda potions and practices were used successfully to replace ineffective antibiotics. The purpose of aromatic plants and oils was not only for medicinal use. The sacred essential oils were believed to be a godly part of nature and played an integral role in the spiritual and philosophical outlook of Ayurvedic medicine, which was holistic at its core.

500 BCE

Around 500 BCE, the **Greeks** recorded knowledge of essential oils, which they adopted from the Egyptians. The

Greek physician Hippocrates (460–377 BCE), known to us as the Father of Medicine, documented the effects of some 300 plants, including thyme, saffron, marjoram, cumin, and peppermint. Hippocrates left a legacy for modern physicians and the medical community. Many doctoral students are administered an amended Hippocratic Oath before the Medical Doctor degree is conferred.

200 BCE

The **Romans** were famous for lavishly applying perfumed oil to their bodies, bedding, and clothes. It was also customary for the Romans to use oils in massages and communal baths.

1000 CE

Essential oils were also of interest in the **Middle East**. Known as the Islamic Golden Age, Avicenna (Abu Ali Sina) lived in Persia during these times and wrote more than 450 books on medicine and healing. Among his interests were herbal remedies and essential oils. He built an essential oil distillery specializing in rose essential oil using the alembic still distillation system, which was created by Cleopatra the Alchemist, an Alexandrian woman of science and philosophy in approximately AD 988.[1]

1096–1291 CE

During the Crusades, the knights and their armies took responsibility for passing on the knowledge of herbal medicines

---

1. Stanton J. Linden. *The Alchemy Reader: From Hermes Trismegistus to Isaac Newton.* Cambridge University Press. 2003. p. 44.

and essential oils they learned from the Arabs. They also returned to Europe with the knowledge of distillation when they transported vats of perfumed oils back to the continent with them. These souvenirs of essential oils, herbs, and spices dramatically changed the face of commerce and trade between Europe and the Middle East.

Middle Ages

In the Middle Ages, oils were extremely popular because the Catholic Church proclaimed that public bathing led to immorality, promiscuous sex, and diseases. Essential oils were used by people to ward off the stench of non-bathing. The Church also forbade the use of herbs as cures for illness because the practice was associated with witches and pagan beliefs. This was a double whammy. The use of essential oils skyrocketed in order to keep the bodily odors in check.

1400–1900 CE

Things changed for herbs and oils in the fifteenth century when **Paracelsus**, also known as Philippus Aureolus Theophrastus Bombastus von Hohenheim, busied himself by exploring the folk remedies and beliefs of the past. He came up with a cure for leprosy using herbal remedies. This discovery commanded serious attention.

Since people hadn't been able to bathe (Can you even imagine this?), and there was new hope for herbal cures, the trade of herbs, spices, and oils increased once again. The Arabs controlled the trade routes, the Dutch became seriously involved in shipping, and Britain formed the East India Trade Company. Huge fortunes were made importing herbs, spices, and oils. The oils were status symbols much like luxury cars are today. The world was changed forever by the plant products of herbs, oils, and spices.

In 1653, **Nicholas Culpeper** wrote *The Complete Herbal*, which still stands as a valuable encyclopedic herbal reference. His book describes many conditions and their herbal remedies that are still effective today. Nothing of much consequence happened in the world of essential oils for close to two centuries thereafter.

Modern Age

Then along came **René-Maurice Gattefossé**, who was born in 1881 and studied to be a chemical engineer by degree. He worked with essential oils in a laboratory partnership with his brother. They created a journal for the elite perfume industry and blended essential oils for the perfume trade in Paris.

In 1918, he came into contact with a liquid cleaner used by hospitals to fight the Spanish flu that was made from essential oils. After clinically noting its effectiveness, he began exploring the antiseptic and medicinal uses for essential oils. He teamed up with doctors in Lyon, France, to research and test the effects of his work and experiments. In 1937, he compiled his findings in the book *Aromathérapie*, which also coined the term "aromatherapy" we use today. Gattefossé was consumed by endless scientific curiosity, and he spent the rest of his life exploring the chemistry and properties of essential oils.

During the 1940s, **Jean Valnet,** a doctor during WWII, studied under Gattefossé. Valnet used essential oils to treat wounded soldiers on the battlefield. He had much success and saved many lives from infection and gangrene.

In the 70s and 80s, essential oils officially came out of hiding, took a public stance, and have not only been used extensively in aromatherapy and massage, but scientists are studying their healing and clinical effects and components around the world. I can't tell you how many scientific and chemistry books I read and researched before writing this book. They all have one big truth in common: they all attest to a grand and strong future for essential oils, medicine, and natural healing. We're on the verge of new and amazing breakthroughs. You're right on schedule by reading this book.

In the next chapter, we'll learn what essential oils are, what they do, where we find them, and how we use them.

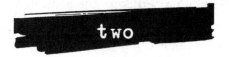

two

What Are Essential Oils?

E ssential oils are the products of plants, bark, leaves, stems, and buds that carry the true *essence* and aroma of the of the originating plant. Hence the term "essential." They aren't really oils at all, but a vital liquid presence living inside plants. They are termed oils because, like oils, these liquids do not mix with water. In chemistry terms, they are aromatic, volatile substances, not that they explode like when we think of a volatile person, but that they give off a scent lasting anywhere from two to twenty-four hours.

We will cover their purposes, how we obtain them, how we use them, and how they work in the body, giving you many examples of why they are such valuable companions in our lives. Essential oils are more than just products of plants. The have healing properties for the body, mind, and soul. Science continues to explore the benefits they have for the physical body and the emotional centers. What follows is a listing and a description of the properties and benefits of essential oils.

What They Do

There are many gifts essential oils possess that are helpful to humans and can accomplish a wide range of tasks using natural properties.

Analgesics

Many essential oils are natural *analgesics,* which means they are substances that affect the nervous system of the body and can subdue pain. Examples include peppermint, lavender, clary sage, Roman chamomile, sandalwood, clove, eucalyptus, and rosemary.

Anti-inflammatory

Many essential oils are *anti-inflammatory*, meaning they can reduce the effects of swelling, redness, and pain at the physical sites of injury, distention, or irritation. Examples include thyme, clove, bergamot, rose, eucalyptus, and lavender.

Antiseptic

Other essential oils have *antiseptic* properties than can help heal infection and microbial invaders. Examples include tea tree, lavender, thyme, eucalyptus, lemon, and sandalwood.

Antifungal

Some are *antifungal* and help prevent the growth of fungi like ringworm, athlete's foot, toenail fungus, tinea versicolor, and jock itch. Thyme, clove, peppermint, tea tree, and eucalyptus are some powerful antifungals and antimicrobials. Be sure to never apply these potent essential oils to your skin directly. Always dilute and use with care.

Antiviral

There are *antiviral* essential oils. Some of these can be antibacterial as well, but definitely can prevent the multiplication and duplication of a viral cell. Examples include tea tree, lemon, peppermint, eucalyptus, and lavender.

Antibacterial

Antibacterial essential oils fight microbes and bacteria that form a single cell in a colony that can invade your body. Examples include thyme, tea tree, rose geranium, and patchouli.

Sedative

There are *sedative* essential oils that can help you calm down or even sleep better. Examples include lavender, frankincense, ylang-ylang, and Roman chamomile.

Energizers

Some are renowned *energizers* and pick-me-ups. Examples include orange, peppermint, eucalyptus, rosemary, thyme, and pine.

Vulnerary

Some are *vulnerary* and can help heal wounds, sores, and prevent tissue degeneration. Examples include bergamot, patchouli, and tea tree. Frankincense works well on scars. Be sure to dilute any of these essential oils before application.

Nervine

Some essential oils promote relaxation because of their *nervine* properties. Use these for headache relief, indigestion, stress, anxiety, tension relief, and anxiety-caused skin rashes and dermatitis. Examples include clary sage, peppermint, rosemary, bergamot, Roman chamomile, sandalwood, and lavender.

Most essential oils are also multi-purpose. Lavender, for example, is a calming essential oil as well as a pain reliever, inflammation soother, antiseptic agent, and a great sleep inducer. In one small bottle you can find many remedies for mind, body, and soul. In part 2 we'll learn more about the properties of twenty essential oils that are perfect for anyone who may be starting out.

How We Obtain Them

We obtain essential oils from plants when we distill them, express them, extract them, or process them under CO_2 pressure. Some processes are done with heat and some are cold. Some use chemicals and solvents, others do not.

Distilled

Lavender, peppermint, tea tree, and eucalyptus are *distilled* because they can withstand the heat and steam caused by boiling water in the alembic still. (Think of a moonshine still as an example.) Originally, the word *distill* emerged from the process of refining alcohol. In the distillation process of heating and steaming, the impurities of a substance are vaporized away. What you have left is the most highly condensed version of the initial liquid or substance. Through the years the word *distill* came to mean the process through which the essence of something is revealed. After distillation, you end up with a product that is the most potent and concentrated version of the original substance.

Expression

Expression takes place via non-heated methods of crushing or pressing the oil out from the hardy peels and stems. Cold-pressed olive oil is obtained this way, and we use the same process for the citrus oils by cold-pressing their peels and rinds to extract the oils.

Extraction

Extraction involves several steps. First, solvents such as petroleum ether, methanol, ethanol, or hexane are used to *extract* the odoriferous lipophilic material from the plant. This is called a *concrete*. A concrete is the concentrated extract that contains the waxes and/or fats as well as the odoriferous material from the plant. The concrete is then doused with alcohol, which extracts the aromatic principle of the material. The final product is known as an *absolute*. Absolutes are primarily used in perfume making.

Carbon Dioxide Pressure

Carbon dioxide is also used under pressure to extract oils and essences from some plants. This is a lower-temperature process and applies only to the processing of those plants that can take the cold and the pressure, like leaves, barks, and woods.

The leftover waters from these distillation processes are called *hydrosols*, less-concentrated liquids, but still bearing the familiar scent of the plant. Hydrosols are used for young children, the elderly, and for aromatic and cosmetic purposes.

Enfleurage

There is another process called *enfleurage,* which is done by placing the petals of oil-rich plants on glass panes covered in animal fat. The oil is slowly leached out of the petals and the spent petals are replaced with new ones until the correct saturation of aroma molecules is achieved. This isn't used much anymore except in the perfume industry because enfleurage requires a lot of time and labor to achieve results.

Forms of Use

You can use essential oils in many ways to improve the condition of your body. The most common ways the body absorbs essential oils are through inhalation (diffusion, inhalers) and application or massage (via the skin organ.)

Diffusers

The aroma of an essential oil (or blend) is distributed into the air and throughout the room/house to provide pleasure, emotional relief, as well as therapeutic assistance. You can disinfect and purify the air based on the different properties you select from each essential oil. You may want to avoid using diffusers that require heat as this method may harm the delicate essential oils. As there is a difference between a humidifier and a diffuser, you'll want to choose a diffuser that uses water or is a cool-based system of distribution. I'll discuss this in greater depth in chapter 26.

Inhalers

These are very personal and portable mini-diffusers of essential oils, which you can make yourself to help and relieve stuffiness, respiration problems, cold symptoms, allergies, smoking cessation, weight control, seasickness, uplifting a mood, or as a source of energy and physical stimulation (more in chapter 26).

Baths

Mix your chosen essential oil(s) with a carrier oil and a proper dispersant in your bath for soothing, relaxing, reviving, calming, and therapeutic benefits. Select the essential oil that features the qualities you want to accomplish in your bath. You must always use a dispersing agent like Solubol or polysorbate to distribute your essential oils into the bath. Otherwise the oils may glob together and potentially harm you or make you very uncomfortable at full potency on your tender skin. See chapter 3 and 4 for more clarity on this topic.

Application

You can use essential oils, always diluted in a carrier oil or dispersant, on your feet, hands, muscles, shoulders, temples, behind the ears, at the wrists, abdomen, chest, lower back, or nape of the neck. Never use them in the ears, eyes, or genitals. If you apply an essential oil to your body and it feels hot, that means it requires more dilution. We will discuss more about safety and precautions in chapter 3 on safety.

Compresses

A compress is a pad of material you apply to the body to stop bleeding or reduce inflammation. For example, you would dilute essential oils using a carrier oil in warm or cool water, submerge a washcloth, and then wring out excess water. You would then apply the compress to the area you want to assist, relieve, cool, or reduce pain.

Massage

Massages are wonderful ways to use essential oils. They are absorbed by the skin and tissues to help relieve pain, tension, and other conditions you may want to improve. Chapter 3 guides you on the safe use of essential oils with a dilution chart. The use of carrier oils paired with your essential oils will be discussed in chapter 4.

Steam Inhalation

This method is used for clearing the sinuses, reducing coughs, clearing congestion, soothing sore throats, and cleaning facial skin. After you boil water and turn off the stove, pour the hot water into a heat-proof basin. Essential oil is added to the hot water with a proper dispersant. You then cover your head with a towel, close your eyes, and, being careful not to burn yourself or your tender skin, inhale the steam for 5–10 minutes.

Face and Body Creams

You can prepare your own cosmetics and body creams using ingredients such as cocoa butter, shea butter, beeswax, and essential oils. The creams can be effective for breakouts, scars, dry skin, wrinkles, and the overall suppleness of your skin. Find recipes in chapter 27.

How Essential Oils Work in the Body

It is vital to understand that when you inhale the aroma from an essential oil, you are actually inhaling molecules. The body intakes essential oils at the atomic level. The topical application of essential oils is also molecular and moves from your skin cells into your muscles, through your bloodstream, and then into the liver and kidneys. As you inhale an essential oil, the scent passes into the bloodstream as molecules; from the lungs it travels to the liver where it is metabolized and filtered. Ninety-five percent of what you inhale is absorbed by the lungs and 5 percent by the brain. From there, the scent molecules travel to the kidneys where they are excreted out of the body.

Here's the great news: essential oils are efficient as they pass through the body. They do not leave long-lasting residue. They do what they were meant to do (i.e., their job) and exit cleanly. The topical application goes from your skin cells into your muscles, into your bloodstream, and then into the liver and kidneys. The liver and kidneys excrete the essential oil molecules and they do not remain in the body for more than a day or two.

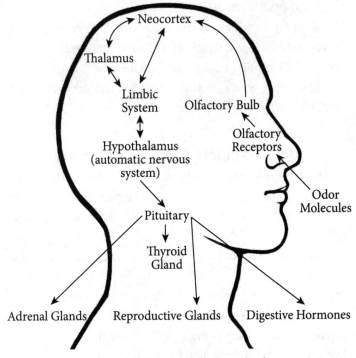

Figure 1: Inhalation of Essential Oils

When you inhale essential oil molecules, your olfactory nerve system identifies the molecules of aroma as pleasant or unpleasant right away. This identification incites memories and feelings.

When the essential oil molecules are absorbed into the cilia, short eyelash-like hairs inside the nostrils, of the olfactory passages, two things occur: there is an immediate (chemical) effect on the brain cells and a subsequent effect on the emotions.

The essential oil is received into the limbic system, which is the center for smell, feelings, emotions, and memory. The limbic system is a complex system of nerves and networks in the brain residing near the edge of the cortex, which is concerned with instinct and mood. It controls the basic emotions (fear, pleasure, anger) and the natural drives (hunger, sex, dominance, care of offspring).

When the limbic system receives input from the olfactory system and essential oils are absorbed into the brain, a psychological impact is created because this is the part of the brain that is associated with feelings and memory. Something like lemon essential oil can lift the spirits and brighten the mood because the brain center recognizes the scent as perky, healthy (growing outdoors), pleasant (in most cases), and invigorating. When you recall the scent of a lemon, you don't see dark colors or feel depressing emotions, do you?

Scents are the closest ties we have to memories. When we recall a memory from the past, we see details and focus on them. When we smell something, our emotional memory is triggered. Our recall is sentient and emotion-based.

Have you ever walked into an open house and smelled fresh bread baking? Didn't it make you feel at home? According to real estate agents, many a house has been sold because the buyer felt an instant sense of recall to happy times and associated that feeling with the property. Emotions influence the decision to purchase.

In the limbic center, the brain triggers signals and sends impulses and instructions to the hypothalamus and the pituitary, which, if you remember from biology class, pretty much rules every function, memory, hormone, and process in the body. It's command central for our bodily functions. Being part of the limbic system, the olfactory bulb has easy access to the amygdala. This is the "fight or flight" reflex center and the seat of emotional memories.

Each essential oil or plant essence is composed of different chemical molecules. Each chemical serves a specific purpose and has a different job assignment. Once the molecules of a given essential oil latches on to the receptors in the body it was specifically designed to help, it gets to work doing the job is was meant to do. Essential oils possess the properties of everything from antibiotic and antimicrobial to anti-inflammatory, vulnerary (wound healing), relaxing, calmative (nervine), and stomachic (assists digestion).

Insert a key in a lock, click, and it opens. You don't have to do a thing: the essential oils are automatically attracted to what needs to be fixed and fix it. It's as if the essential oil is already pre-programmed with its assignment. It does the same thing with the plant it came from. It protects them from the inside out. So, too, with humans. Our job is to select the essential oil that is pre-designed for the healing we need. Then dilute it and apply it, inhale it, or use it in whatever manner is suitable for the condition we want to fix.

We let the essential oil go to work, do its job, and we are on our way to improving body, mind, and soul. That's why essential oils are nature's gifts to us.

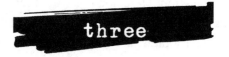

three

Safety and Guidelines for Using Essential Oils

It's easy to become enthusiastic about using essential oils; they are enticing, aromatic, and extremely appealing. I got very excited about them initially, and, back when I was a beginner, I learned some lessons the hard way. It never occurred to me that essential oils needed to be diluted. I mean, why would they? They are natural compounds and Mother Nature wouldn't hurt us, would she?

After my first encounter with red skin and a visible trace of an all-too-potent essential oil, I did my research. I was shocked to learn how potent essential oils really are and, after learning more about them, it began to make sense. I know reading directions and manuals is not very exciting, but I implore you to read this chapter thoroughly for your own safety and protection. Here you'll get the basics on which types of oils are best to use, how to go about safely diluting them, when you shouldn't use certain oils, how to safely dispose of expired oils, and more.

Buy Organic, 100% Pure, or Wildcrafted

Out in the wild and wooly marketplace there is a huge debate about the labeling and use of essential oils. There are so many competing brands, types, blends, and creative labeling that it's hard to know which is which. The second most frequent question I get asked by my students is what brand to buy. My opinion is based on two facts: first, essential oils are extremely condensed after processing, so you get a very potent product in a very small bottle. Second, you put these essential oils into your body via inhalation, or onto your body via massage or application. It stands to reason that if these essential oils are condensed to their most potent state, then so are any toxins or contaminates that were on the plant when it was harvested and processed. The toxins and contaminates would also be powerfully condensed, and we do not want to have highly concentrated poisons, toxins, and pollutants in our body or on our skin.

The reason is simple: essential oils pass through the organs of the body via the lungs, liver, kidney, brain, and bloodstream, and you don't want any toxins, chemicals, fertilizers, preservatives, or growth hormones traveling through your precious body. Toxins can occur during planting, harvesting, and extraction. Toxin-free essential oils are the only ones you want to put on or in your body via massage, application, or inhalation.

The best way to prevent the unwanted contaminates in our essential oil products is to purchase only those essential oils labeled as organic, 100 percent pure, or wildcrafted. Avoid words like "therapeutic grade," "pharmaceutical grade," "natural," "100 percent natural," "clinical," and "purest." That's usually marketing mumbo jumbo. You want to make sure the essential oils you buy are wildcrafted, 100 percent pure, or organic.

Organic, 100 percent pure, or wildcrafted essential oils are the purest and most condensed oils available in the world. When we hold our essential oils in high regard and have respect for them, we will naturally treat them as the special creations they are. Be sure to refresh your memory with the properties, benefits, and uses of each essential oil you intend to use, and make note of its proprietary cautions (we'll get to that in part 2).

Never Use Essential Oils Neat

Always dilute essential oils. No exceptions. Unless you are working with a certified Aromatherapist, don't gamble with this. You'll hear people say that you can use lavender, tea tree, or chamomile *neat*, which means undiluted. Don't risk it. Always dilute and do a patch test before you use any essential oil. (We'll get into an explanation of the patch test later in this chapter.) This way you can avoid unintended consequences such as sensitization or burns.

You need to dilute your essential oils with a carrier oil. You want to choose carrier oils that you like and that suit your dilution purposes. Some carrier oils are great for skin and for massage, others are better for wrinkles and sensitive skin. See the expanded explanation in chapter 4 on carrier oils. Select a few that can serve your multiple purposes. Keep them in a cool dark place, or maybe even refrigerate them for longer shelf life. Never store them in the kitchen or confuse them for cooking oils. If you live with others who might mistake them for something to fry an egg in, use a label to make sure they know it's for essential oil purposes only, not cooking.

Dilution Guidelines

Essential oils are the aromatic fluids that help protect the plant from invaders, parasites, insects, fungus, and bacteria. If they can do all that for the plant, imagine what they can do for us. Especially considering that we extract the fluids and distill or press them down to make a condensed concentration that is exponentially more powerful than how they exist in the plant. With this in mind, it's important to remember that one of the biggest mistakes we can make using essential oils is to not dilute them properly. Diluting essential oils is very important for two main safety reasons:

1. To avoid reactions such as skin irritation, sensitization, and phototoxicity. These are temporary and visible, but in extreme cases can cause permanent damage. I'll explain more in a moment.

2. To avoid systemic toxicity, such as fetotoxicity, poisoning or harming a fetus; hepatoxicity, chemical liver impairment; carcinogenicity, a substance that

promotes cancer cell growth; and neurotoxicity, a chemical that causes adverse effects on the central nervous system, dilute your essential oils. Systemic toxicities may not be reversible. These conditions can result from ingesting essential oils or putting them on your body without the proper dilution. Going into the sun with a phototoxic essential oil on your skin can cause burns to the skin. The ultraviolet rays of the sun increase the potency of the essential oil, which can result in unfavorable chemical reactions.

Sensitization means that you can develop a lifelong sensitivity to a particular essential oil that, in the most severe circumstances, can cause a reaction from a simple reddening of the skin or rash to anaphylactic shock, respiratory problems, or severe skin reactions. Sensitization can be permanent and cause a reaction even when you are in close proximity to the essential oil. For example, many common household products contain lavender essential oil and, if overused or not properly diluted, can cause you to have permanent allergic reactions to body soaps, laundry detergents, room sprays, and cleaning products that contain the lavender scent for the rest of your life. It is advisable to dilute every essential oil to prevent sensitization in the first place.

A good rule of thumb to follow for essential oils is: *less is more* when using them. If a recipe or dilution calls for a certain number of drops, follow that guideline. Do not add more just because you think it will work or smell better. In many cases the less you use, the more powerful the result.

Children and elderly people require a greater dilution than people ages eighteen to sixty. Follow the age-appropriate dilution ratios for safety. The percentage of dilution depends on the results you are trying to achieve. Follow these tips when diluting essential oils:

For Children

- .25 percent dilution (one drop per four teaspoons of carrier oil)—for children between three months and two years. It is recommended you only use essential oils on children under the proper supervision of an Aromatherapist. For children under two, it is best to use hydrosols instead. Hydrosols—also known as floral waters, hydroflorates, flower waters, or distillates—are products obtained from the process of steam distilling plant materials. Hydrosols are like essential oils but in a far less potent, more watery concentration. To make an easy dilution of this strength, follow the chart directions for 1 percent dilution and then dilute that mixture by adding three more teaspoons of carrier oil to the blend.

- 1–2 percent dilution—for children from age two to six years; pregnant women (of acceptable oils); elderly adults; those with sensitive skin, compromised immune systems, or other serious health issues. This is also the dilution to use for massaging a large area of the body.

- 2–3 percent dilution—for children ages six to fifteen years. Use the lower dilution for the youngest age and progress in strength as the child ages.

For Adults

- 2–3 percent dilution—ideal for most adults and in most situations. This is also the recommended dilution for daily skin care.

- 3–10 percent dilution—best used short-term for a temporary health issue, such as a muscle injury, bruising, wound healing, or respiratory congestion. Up to 10 percent dilution is considered for critical care and only used for a short time, no more than two to three days.

- 25 percent dilution (25 drops per teaspoon of carrier oil; 125–150 drops per ounce). On special occasions, a dilution of this strength may be warranted. Examples include severe muscle cramping, bad bruising, or intense pain. Always consult a certified Aromatherapist for stronger dilutions.

For Seniors

- Use the same dilutions for children under the age of six, because elderly folks have sensitive skin and are very reactive to essential oils. Always use a mild dilution.

Overall Tip

- Always use the lowest dilution of essential oils possible that will give you the most effective results.

Dilution	1%	2%	3%	5%	10%	25%
EO drops per 1 tsp. carrier oil	1	2	3	5	10	25
EO drops per 2 tsp. carrier oil	2	4	6	10	20	50
EO drops per 3 tsp. carrier oil	3	6	9	15	30	75
EO drops per 4 tsp. carrier oil	4	8	12	20	40	100
EO drops per 5 tsp. carrier oil	5	10	15	25	50	125
EO drops per 6 tsp. carrier oil	6	12	18	30	60	150

Figure 2: Dilution Chart

Tips for Essential Oil Measurements

Essential oils are usually sold in 5-ml, 10-ml, and 15-ml dark glass bottles. You can purchase them in 1-ounce, 2-ounce, 4-ounce, and up in sizes if you are buying in bulk. The 5-ml bottle holds approximately 75 drops of oil. The 10-ml bottle holds about 175 drops of oil, and the 15-ml bottle holds around 250 drops. The thicker essential oils like patchouli and sandalwood may have a few less drops in the bottle due to their viscosity. The orifice reducer at the top of the bottle is put in place to allow only a drop or two to be released at a time for your protection. This will help as you measure things for mixes and dilutions.

When diluting your oils, it is helpful to have a conversion reference handy. Here is a list for various measurement equivalents:

100 drops = 1 tsp. = 5 ml = ⅙ oz.

200 drops = 2 tsp. = 10 ml = ⅓ oz.

300 drops = 3 tsp. = 15 ml = ⅙ oz.

400 drops = 4 tsp. = 20 ml = ⅔ oz.

500 drops = 5 tsp. = 25 ml = ⅚ oz.

600 drops = 6 tsp. = 30 ml = 1 oz.

Patch Test Instruction

Conduct a patch test on yourself and others so you do not cause a rash or other problem. You want to avoid sensitization at all cost. Sensitization occurs when you have too much of a good thing. Your body can react with an allergic reaction from an itch to a full-body rash to anaphylactic shock. Think of poison ivy. When the oil in the leaf contacts your skin, it produces welts. That's the extreme. Once you are sensitized to an aroma or oil, it may or may not be a problem for you for the rest of your life. You cannot reverse sensitization, so be sure you don't cause it in the first place. The patch test is your best way to figure out if you are allergic to or have an adverse reaction to any of the essential oils. It takes an hour or more to conduct the patch test, but if you are patient and follow the patch test protocol below, you may save yourself a lifetime of discomfort.

Adverse reactions you might experience from essential oils include:

- A red rash or raised bumps on the skin
- Hives
- Itching ranging from moderate to severe
- Dry or cracked and scaly skin

- Blisters, crusting, and weeping sores
- Swelling and tenderness
- Painful burning
- Shortness of breath
- Anaphylactic shock is an extremely rare reaction, but it is a possibility

Patch Test Steps

Open the essential oil bottle. Open a carrier oil bottle. Have them both available in your test area.

Gently dip a toothpick into the essential oil bottle and extract a small drop of the oil. (Have a bottle of olive oil standing by. Olive oil will be used to immediately wipe the essential oil off your hand or arm if there is a reaction. Do not use soap and water as it will not eradicate the oil from your skin.)

Mix the essential oil with one or two drops of a carrier oil.

Drop the essential oil and carrier oil mix onto your arm or leg and observe how your skin reacts. If there is a negative reaction of any kind, immediately cleanse the area with olive oil to wipe away the essential oil. There are a couple of reasons why you might have a reaction. One is that you are allergic to the essential oil and its chemical components. The other is that there are toxins, pesticides, or other impurities in the essential oil.

If you do not have an immediate reaction to the essential oil mix, place a drop on the inside of your elbow, cover it with a Band-Aid, and leave it on for twenty-four hours. After twenty-four hours, remove the bandage and see if there is any kind of a reaction. Do not proceed with use if there is a reaction.

You might feel like this is overkill or unnecessary, but it isn't. I want to share with you an anecdote of an adverse reaction to an essential oil after not first patch testing.

One woman loved the smell of lavender so much she rubbed it neat on her face and arms at bedtime so she could smell it during the night. She woke up red-skinned and so stuffed up that she could barely breathe. She discovered that she was allergic to lavender essences and now she can't even be in the same room as lavender hand cream, lest she react with shortness of breath. She has to stay away from fabric softener dryer sheets, lavender detergents, lavender room sprays, or anything with lavender in it or she feels the reaction. It is interesting to note that some hotel laundries innocently use lavender in their laundry and cleaning procedures.

Don't Use in These Areas or Circumstances

Avoid using near eyes, ears, or genitals. These are areas where the skin is tender (there are some rare exceptions in high dilution). Never ingest essential oils. Never use in the eyes, ears, internally, or through injection or IV. You'd be surprised at how many people think this is a good idea.

Never take essential oils internally! The only exception is if you are under the supervision of a certified Aromatherapist, not someone who took a weekend online course and earned a downloadable certificate. Be sure you intake the essential oils only under proper supervision. Many people have incurred permanent internal and chronic conditions from unsupervised internal consumption. A certified Aromatherapist has spent at least 150–200 hours studying and learning about essential oils, their content, chemistry, human physiology, uses, and safety from a credential aromatherapy school and has clinical experience properly working with essential oils and clients. Remember, ingesting any essential oils could result in permanent impairment or death.

Caution should also be applied when using with children, those who are pregnant, and those with existing conditions (we'll get more into those specific cautions later in this chapter). Further on in the book there may be a couple of exceptions to these rules, but they will follow an exact recipe, instruction, and dilution.

Using Oils with Water

Essential oils do not mix with water. The oil rises to the top because it is less dense than water. For baths and steaming, you want to use the correct dispersant so the oil molecules are evenly distributed and do not stay globed together. This concentration can result in injury. Do not try to wipe off essential oils with soap and water. The water will not disperse the oils. Instead, use another type of oil, like olive, to remove the essential oil from your hands or skin.

When steam inhaling essential oils, make sure they are diluted and properly dispersed in steaming water: turn the heat off, cover your head, and close your eyes to avoid heat or steam from damaging your eyes.

We will get more into using dispersants with your oils in water in chapter 4.

Photosensitivity

There are some essential oils that are phototoxic and should not be used if you are going out into the sunlight, using tanning beds, or will subject yourself to ultraviolet rays within twelve to eighteen hours of using phototoxic essential oils. Skin damage results when particular chemicals, furocoumarins (FCs), in the essential oils react when exposed to ultraviolet light.

Do not use citrus oils on your skin or in lotions if they are applied in the morning as photosensitivity may occur from exposure to the sun. The citrus essential oils not regarded as photosensitive are: red mandarin (*Citrus nobilis*), sweet orange (*Citrus sinensis*), tangerine (*Citrus reticulata*), and blood orange (*Citrus x sinensis*).

Phototoxic essential oils include (those from the list of 20 in this book are in bold):

- Angelica root *(Angelica glauca)*
- **Bergamot (*Citrus bergamia*)**
- Cumin *(Cuminum cyminum)*
- Expressed bitter orange *(Citrus x aurantium)*
- Expressed grapefruit *(Citrus paradisi)*
- **Expressed lemon (*Citrus limon*)**
- Expressed lime *(Citrus aurantifolia)*
- Fig leaf absolute *(Ficus carica)*
- Lemon verbena *(Aloysia triphylla)*
- Mandarin leaf *(Citrus reticulata)*
- Orange, bitter *(Citrus x aurantium)*
- Rue *(Ruta graveolens)*
- Tagetes (*Tagetes minuta*)

I was doing a book signing when a lovely young woman asked me if I could recommend an essential oil to heal a chemical burn on her neck. It turned out it was caused by bergamot. She had applied some before a beach yoga class. By the end of class, she had some reddening and washed it off with soap and water when she got home. Needless to say, it was all a bad mix.

I advised her not to try to fix the burn with essential oils. It would fade in time, but if she wanted a faster remedy it might involve some laser work like the kind used for removing a tattoo. I recommended she see a dermatologist.

Another strange occurrence is a syndrome called "margarita burn." This happens when bartenders who work on the beach or poolside, like at a tropical resort, handle fresh limes and squeeze the rinds all day long in the sun for fancy drinks, beer, and shots of tequila. The oils of the limes get onto their hands. The sun's rays burn into the oils and suddenly you have *phytophotodermatitis. Phyto*, meaning from the plant, and *photo*, meaning from the sun's UV rays.

Highly Toxic Essential Oils

The following is a list of essential oils that are toxic and should never be used by a consumer unless under the guidance and supervision of a certified Aromatherapist. None of the twenty oils from this book appear in this list.

- Ajowan (*Trachyspermum capticum*)
- Arnica (*Arnica montana*)
- Bitter Almond (*Prunus amygdalus var. amara*)
- Birch (*Betula*)

- Boldo Leaf (*Peumus boldus*)
- Calamus (*Acorus calamus*)
- Camphor (*Cinnamomum camphora*)
- Cassia (*Cinnamomum cassia*)
- Deertongue (*Carphephorus Odoratissimus*)
- Garlic (*Allium sativum*)
- Horseradish (*Cochlearia armoracia*)
- Jaborandi (*Pilocarpus jaborandi*)
- Melilotus (*Melilotus officialnalis*)
- Mugwort (*Artemisia vulgaris*)
- Mustard (*Brassica nigra*)
- Onion (*Allium cepa*)
- Rue (*Ruta graveolens*)
- Sassafras (*Sassafras albidum*)
- Savin (*Juniperus sabina*)
- Tansy (*Tanacetum vulgare*)
- Thuja (*Thuja occidentalis*)
- Wintergreen (*Gaultheria procumbens*)
- Wormseed (*Chenopodium ambrosioides*)
- Wormwood (*Artemisia absinthium*)

Pregnancy Cautions

Pregnant women can use some essential oils. If you are pregnant or nursing, consult a qualified Aromatherapist for the suitability and safety of specific oils. Many essential oils should not be used during pregnancy; some only need to be avoided for the first three to four months; others may be helpful during labor, but may otherwise pose a threat to you and the fetus. Seek professional help before using, and read the information for each essential oil for the suggested times for use or non-use of these pregnancy-sensitive essential oils.

Below is a list of essential oils to avoid or modify if you are pregnant or breastfeeding. Those from the list of twenty in this book are in bold.

- Aniseed (*Pimpinella anisum*)
- Basil (*Ocimum basilicum*)
- **Bergamot** (*Citrus bergamia*)
- Birch (*Betula*)
- Camphor (*Cinnamomum camphora*)
- **Clove** (*Syzygium aromaticum*)
- **Frankincense** (*Boswellia carteri*)
- Hyssop (*Hyssopus officinalis*)
- **Melissa** (*Melissa officinalis*)
- Mugwort (*Artemisia vulgaris*)
- Parsley (*Petroselinum sativum*)
- Pennyroyal (*Mentha pulegium*)
- **Peppermint** (*Mentha x piperita*)
- **Roman chamomile** (*Chamaemelum nobile*)
- **Rose geranium** (*Pelargonium graveolens*)
- **Rosemary** (*Rosmarinus officinalis*)
- Sage (*Salvia officinalis*)
- Tansy (*Tanacetum vulgare*)
- Tarragon (*Artemisia dracunculus*)
- Thuja (*Thuja occidentalis*)

- **Thyme** *(Thymus vulgaris)*
- Wintergreen (*Gaultheria procumbens*)
- Wormwood (*Artemisia absinthium*)
- **Ylang-ylang** *(Cananga odorata)*

You can check out additional safety issue details for using essential oils during pregnancy in the back of the book under Recommended Resources.

Caution with Other Existing Conditions

If you have a serious medical condition, such as (but not limited to) high blood pressure, heart disease, kidney or liver disease, cancer, thrombosis, varicose veins, mental illness, or epilepsy, consult a qualified Aromatherapist and a medical doctor for professional advice on recommended oils and dosages. Take extra caution when using on people undergoing chemotherapy or psychiatric treatments and the elderly.

If you are taking medications for a serious medical condition, there can be interactions with essential oils. Please consult a qualified Aromatherapist and your medical doctor before engaging in the use of essential oils. Many physicians are not familiar with the benefits of essential oils, so please reach out to one that considers them a useful alternative therapy.

Caution with Children

Do not use on infants or premature babies. Skin application and direct inhalations should be avoided for children under five years old. The dilution chart is very specific about how much you can use, or how much and how long you can diffuse certain essential oils on and around infants and children.

Do not use peppermint essential oil on children under five years old. Peppermint has high percentages of menthol, which can cause apnea and bronchial spasms when inhaled or massaged.

When preparing a blend for a child, remember that you will halve the strength—where you would normally include a 2 percent dilution of essential oil to the carrier oil, you will prepare a 1 percent dilution for use on a child.

If you are using a diffusion blend with children, do not leave them unattended with the diffuser at any time, and only diffuse for one to two minutes per session with children under twelve years of age.

Below is a list of essential oils to *not* use on children without the advice of a qualified Aromatherapist. Those from the list of twenty in this book are in bold.

- Basil *(Ocimum basilicum)*
- Bay *(Laurus nobilis)*
- Benzoin *(Styrax benzoin)*
- **Bergamot *(Citrus bergamia)***
- Birch *(Betula)*
- Black pepper *(Piper nigrum)*
- Cassia *(Cinnamomum cassia)*
- Cedarwood *(Cedrus atlantica)*
- Cinnamon Bark *(Cinnamomum verum)*
- *Cinnamon Leaf (Cinnamomum zeylanicum)*
- Citronella *(Cymbopogon nardus)*

- **Clove** *(Syzygium aromaticum)*
- Costus *(Saussurea costus)*
- Cumin *(Cuminum cyminum)*
- Elecampane *(Inula helenium)*
- **Eucalyptus globulus** *(Eucalyptus globulus)*
- Fennel *(Foeniculum vulgare)*
- Fir *(Abies)*
- Ginger *(Zingiber officinale)*
- Helichrysum *(Helichrysum italicum)*
- Juniper *(Juniperus)*
- **Lemon** *(Citrus × limon)*
- Lemon verbena *(Aloysia citrodora)*
- Lemongrass *(Cymbopogon)*
- **Melissa** *(Melissa officinalis)*
- Nutmeg *(Myristica fragrans)*
- Oak moss *(Evernia prunastri)*
- **Orange** *(Citrus × sinensis)*
- Oregano *(Origanum vulgare)*
- Parsley seed *(Petroselinum crispum)*
- **Peppermint** *(Mentha × piperita)*
- Pimento berry *(Pimenta dioica)* (Allspice)
- **Pine** *(Pinus)*
- Tagetes *(Tagetes minuta)*
- **Thyme (red)** *(Thymus vulgaris)*

Caution with Pets

Essential oils should not be used on animals unless you're working with a trained Aromatherapist who specializes in using essential oils on animals and your veterinarian. According to Aromatherapist and Animal Specialist Kelly Holland Azzaro,[2] some animals respond to spot treatments of certain essential oils, hoof care, and massage therapy. Cats are not among these animals that can tolerate the use of essential oils. Their systems are too fragile and cannot break down the chemical substances found in essential oils. Nor can fish, reptiles, birds, rodents, gerbils, hamsters, rabbits, guinea pigs, chinchillas, etc. See the Recommended Resources section in the back of the book for more information on animal safety with essential oils.

Exposure

We never want to take essential oils for granted. They require special attention when we are working with them, blending them, or making personal products. Here are some additional things to think about before working with your essential oils.

Do not prepare formulations in outdoor locations or in sunshine. The UV rays can damage the essential oils and shorten the life of carrier oils.

Do not expose children under twelve to any more than one to two minutes of diffused essential oils.

---

2. Azzaro, Kelly Holland. "Animal Aromatherapy and Essential Oil Safety," https://naha.org/assets/uploads/Animal_Aromatherapy_Safety_NAHA.pdf.

Never leave essential oil bottles open to the air. Close them tightly and store them in a dark, cool place in dark glass bottles.

If you buy essential oils in large bottles or bulk, make sure you decant them into smaller bottles after you use half the contents of the larger essential oil bottle. Too much oxygen in the half-filled bottle can accelerate rancidity and oxidation.

Shelf Life and Storage

Keep essential oils away from flames and electrical outlets /sources. Store them in dark bottles, in a cool, dry place, and safely secured away from young children, guests, housekeepers, babysitters, and pets.

Essential oils do not contain water and they do not grow mold, mildew, or yeast due to the antibacterial and antiviral properties they contain. But they do change over time, and some can turn rancid and spoil. Several things can affect the shelf life of essential oils and can cause them to lose their freshness: light, heat, air (oxygen), moisture, and time.

1–2 Years

Essential oils that have a higher quantity of monoterpenes or oxides have the shortest shelf life—approximately one to two years. Limonene is found in bergamot, lemon, and orange. Pinene is found in eucalyptus, pine, and rosemary.

2–3 Years

Essential oils that have a higher quantity of phenols may last up to three years. Clove, thyme.

4–5 Years

Essential oils that contain ketones, monoterpenols, and/or esters have a shelf life of approximately four to five years. Frankincense, peppermint, rosemary.

6 years

Essential oils with a higher amount of sesquiterpenes and sesquiterpenols can last up to six years. Lavender, clary sage, Roman chamomile, patchouli, lemon.

Exceptions to this rule are patchouli, sandalwood, and ylang-ylang, which do not spoil over time if stored correctly, and can actually improve with age.

Spillage

Avoid spilling on furniture and appliances. Essential oil spillage can ruin a finish, bubble latex paint, and eat away the surface of things like your cellphone, plastic keyboard, Styrofoam, plastic bottles, and more.

Disposal

You will need to dispose of old, rancid, or foul-smelling essential oils in a way that is compatible with safety considerations as well as local regulations and green protocol. Some essential oils come with an MSDS, a Material Safety Data Sheet, which is a document that details flammability, health hazards, first-aid procedures, and disposal information for chemicals. The manufacturer or bottler can supply you with such data or you can research the data on the internet. Your local sanitation company can direct you to the safe procedures. Do not pour essential oils down the drain as they can leech into public waterways and out to sea, which can contaminate and poison sea creatures and wildlife. Essential oils are also flammable and can be set on fire, causing danger and damage to the environment and structures. Use care.

You can use aged essential oils, or ones that are past their use-by dates on dryer sheets, in the laundry, and a few drops down the drain to freshen it, but not an entire bottle.

Some online advisors suggest you dig a hole in your garden or lawn and pour old oil there. This is not a good idea because pets, wildlife, and the roots of your plants and grass may be damaged when coming into contact with these potent essential oils. Always stay environmentally aware when disposing of essential oils.

If the essential oils are not too old, you can use them in diffusers for aromatherapy purposes. They can also be used to freshen diaper pails or in garbage cans.

Another way to dispose of essential oils is to place a bowl of baking soda in your garage or shed, dump your expired essential oils into it, and let them evaporate. Be sure you keep this mixture out of reach of small children or pets.

You can also bring old oils to your local hazardous waste site, the same place you take old paint and chemicals.

Yet another way is to purchase a bag of sand and have it on hand. You can empty your bottle of essential oils into the sand and seal it in an airtight jar or Tupperware container and take to a recycling location for proper disposal. This is my favorite way to dispose of them. You can also seek information from the EPA or your local Waste Management Department of your region, community, city, or country.

Remember, essential oils are hazardous materials that are in the same category as pharmaceuticals, paint thinners, chemicals, gasoline, and fuels. You cannot dump essential oils in your garbage can or flush them down the drain any more than you can dump old medications or paint thinner down the drain or toilet. As a result of past misuse, there are standards in place for proper disposal that protect our ground water, water systems, oceans, ponds, rivers, pets, and wildlife.

For additional safety information you can refer to the National Association for Holistic Aromatherapy (NAHA). See the Recommended Resources section for more on this subject.

Finding an Aromatherapist or Healthcare Practitioner

Taking care of yourself and being proactive with alternative therapies is a positive thing to do. But, if your symptoms persist or are recurrent, or if you suffer from a serious medical condition or are taking prescription drugs, I recommend you consult both a medical doctor and a qualified Aromatherapist before attempting to help yourself. Many naturopaths, chiropractors, and osteopaths are certified Aromatherapists, too. Check their essential oils educational qualifications. NAHA. org provides a list of authorized schools for certification. (See the Recommended Resources section in the back of the book.) The ideal is to find a practitioner as well as a doctor you trust and who are prepared to work together with you to explore natural health alternatives.

I recommend you read about the properties of the essential oils in part 2 before you rush out and buy a whole slew of them, so you can decide which ones you want to buy first. There are hundreds available, but you may want to start selectively, otherwise you can blow a whole month's rent on oils you may not even want or need once you learn more about them. (Experience is a wonderful teacher and I am passing along a few lessons to you that I learned the hard way. You're welcome!) Before we get into those distinct oils, we will look at choosing and buying carrier oils and how to mix your essential oils with your carrier oils and dispersants safely and properly.

four

Pairing Carrier Oils and Dispersants with Your Essential Oils

Dilution is one of the first things a beginner learns. It is the key to using essential oils correctly and safely. In my beginner classes, one of the first questions is "Why do we have to dilute?" We answered the safety issues in the last chapter, and now we can move on to some wonderful carrier oils that bring their own personalities and properties into the mix. We dilute because we want to use the correct amount of essential oils for the problem we want to solve or the issue we want to alleviate. Carrier oils are a world unto themselves. Here's a list of some of the ones I enjoy working with, and why.

Favorite Carrier Oils

The following are some of my favorite carrier oils.

Apricot Kernel Oil

Contains oleic acid and linoleic acid and is antibacterial. Because of superior absorption and softening properties, it's great for face, skin, hair, eczema, psoriasis, and dermatitis.

Argan Oil

High in vitamin E, it has the aroma of hazelnut and helps with antiaging and preserves skin elasticity.

Avocado Oil

Consists of oleic acid, a monounsaturated omega-9 fatty acid, which is good for penetrating, rejuvenating, and moisturizing skin.

Black Seed Oil (source: black cumin)

Contains linoleic acid; omega-6 fatty acids; vitamins A, B_1, B_2, D, and E; potassium; calcium; phosphorous; magnesium; sodium; and copper. It is antifungal, antibiotic, analgesic, anti-inflammatory, and good for hair and skin while boasting a long shelf life.

Borage Seed Oil

Highest-known source for GLA (gamma linoleic acid), it is anti-inflammatory and anti-thrombotic. (Do not use during pregnancy or right before or after surgery, as it thins the blood.) Good for eczema, rheumatism, stretch marks, wrinkles, and arthritis. Combine with sweet almond oil for best results.

Carrot Seed Oil

Antibacterial with vitamin A and beta-carotene. High in minerals, it is helpful for antiaging skin products.

Coconut Oil

Contains highly saturated fats. Antibacterial qualities fight microbes, but since it is high in saturated fats, I only recommend it for hair use.

Emu Oil

High in omega-3, omega-6, and omega-9 fatty acids and antioxidants. Emu oil has analgesic and anti-inflammatory properties. Good for joint pain, wound healing, and skin repair.

Evening Primrose Oil

Rich source of omega-6 essential fatty acids, and vitamin E. Evening primrose oil contains linoleic acid as well as GLA. It's anti-inflammatory, is good for skin, wound healing, acne, psoriasis, and eczema. Evening primrose oil can act as a blood thinner, so be careful when using it if you're also taking blood-thinning medications.

Flaxseed Oil

Contains alpha-linolenic acid (ALA), a form of omega-3 fatty acid, and is a powerful anti-inflammatory. Good for joints, eczema, and psoriasis.

Grape Seed Oil

Contains vitamin E and phenolic antioxidants and is a rich source of omega-6 fatty acids. Good for skin, acne, scars, stretch marks, and is hypoallergenic with a long shelf life.

Hazelnut Oil
Rich in vitamins B_1, B_6, E, niacin, folic acid, magnesium, and potassium, and it has astringent qualities that help clear up acne.

Hemp Seed Oil
Rich in omega-6 and omega-3 polyunsaturated fatty acids. The analgesic qualities assist with muscle and joint pain. Good for skin and eczema. Does not contain CBD or THC.

Jojoba Oil
Contains vitamin E, vitamin B complex, silicon, chromium, copper, and zinc. It has a high percentage of iodine for healing. It is anti-inflammatory and good for joints. Also good for skin, acne, hair, and scalp dryness. Buy unrefined for non-greasy feel.

Kukui Nut Oil
Vitamins A, C, and E, plus antioxidants from the candlenut tree. Light oil, good for psoriasis, eczema, aging skin, and acne, but has a shorter shelf life.

Macadamia Nut Oil
Contains niacin, calcium, iron, magnesium, phosphorous, potassium, sodium, copper, omega-9s, and antioxidants. Good for nourishing and protecting skin, especially mature or aging skin.

Neem Oil
Contains vitamin E and is good for skin and hair. It also contains azadirachtin, an active component for repelling bugs

and killing pests like lice. Good for inflammation and skin care because it stimulates collagen production.

Olive Oil
Contains large amounts of antioxidants, is antibacterial, and contains vitamin K. It's also good for inflammation and skin care. Helps with sprain relief and bruise care.

Pomegranate Oil
Contains punicic acid, an omega-5 fatty acid, with strong anti-inflammatory benefits. Good for skin and acne because it balances skin pH.

Rose Hip Oil
Contains vitamin A, antioxidants, and fatty acids. Good for skin, acne, eczema, burns, and antiaging, as well as helping to lighten and restore suppleness to skin.

Safflower Oil
Rich in the essential omega-6 fatty acid linoleic acid and is high in vitamin E, which is good for skin and acne.

Sesame Oil
Natural antibacterial, antiviral, and antioxidant properties; contains vitamins A, B, and E, as well as calcium, magnesium, and phosphorous. Good for skin and hair, and inhibits premature graying, skin aging, and rheumatism in joints.

Soybean Oil
Contains vitamin E, lecithin, and anti-oxidants, which make it a great anti-wrinkle and antiaging oil. Light and thin oil for easy absorption.

Sunflower Oil
Contains palmitic acid, stearic acid, oleic acid, lecithin, carotenoids, selenium, calcium, zinc, potassium, iron, and linoleic acid, plus vitamins A, D, and E. Good for skin and is anti-inflammatory, odorless, and doesn't stain.

Sweet Almond Oil
Contains vitamins A, B_1, B_2, B_6, E, monosaturated fatty acids, protein, potassium, and zinc. Light oil that is good for skin, dermatitis, psoriasis, eczema, hair, and massage.

Tamanu Oil
Antibacterial with properties for tissue and cell rejuvenation for the skin, topical infections (yeast), scars, eczema, and psoriasis.

Wheat Germ Oil
Is thick and viscous. Good for the skin and antiaging. Contains vitamins A, B_1, B_2, B_6, E, F, magnesium, zinc, and iron. Helps dry skin, achy muscles, and aging and mature skin.

Choosing and Buying
I found I most liked working with the carrier oils in the list above, though it's all based on personal preference. Some of you may prefer the aroma of the nut oils and others may enjoy a more herbal scent. There are many more on the market you can choose as well. Please experiment with your own carrier oils and find the one or two you enjoy most. Choose one that you like the texture and smell of. I usually have ten to twelve on hand for cosmetic projects and personal use.

Be sure to research the properties a carrier oil possesses before you buy it. Carrier oils can enhance the therapeutic value of the essential oils you are using, especially if they have qualities that complement the essential oil, like being antibacterial, antifungal, anti-inflammatory, or are loaded with vitamins and minerals for the skin. Be sure you buy high-quality carrier oils from reputable merchants and store them away from heat, light, and high temperatures. Cooler storage is best for their longest life and best performance. I try not to order any essential oils or carrier oils when the temperatures outside are high since delivered packages can be left in the mailbox or on the porch. These delicate oils can be damaged by excess heat and their longevity affected. The same can be said of freezing temperatures. I limit my ordering to the more temperate months of spring and fall when I order online.

Always buy carrier oils cold-pressed, no additives, no fragrances, 100 percent pure, organic, wildcrafted, non-GMO, and rich in fatty acids. Be sure to find pure and organic carrier oils, just like the essential oils you buy. Buy them unrefined, raw, and organic. Many carrier oils are mixed with cheaper, unhealthy vegetable oils. Read the labels and avoid ones that contain anything but the real deal. Look in your local health food store for carrier oils that meet these guidelines.

Toss your carrier oil if it is cloudy, has a foul odor, smells rancid or off, or feels gummy in your fingers. Please remember to store them in a cool, dry, dark place. I use a small refrigerator in the garage for my essential oils and carrier oils storage, away from people, pets, and curious kids.

Best Carrier Oils for a Specific
Purpose or Condition

Acne

Best carrier oils for acne include black seed, apricot kernel, jojoba, sesame seed, coconut, and sweet almond. Nut and seed oils are great, and with stearic acid they have anti-inflammatory and antibacterial qualities to help with acne.

Antiaging

Best carrier oils for antiaging include wheat germ, jojoba, rose hip, argan, borage, macadamia nut, olive, neem, and tamanu.

Burns

Best carrier oil for burns include rose hip, emu, and shea butter.

Face/Creams

Best carrier oils for face creams include apricot kernel, carrot seed, pomegranate, neem, and tamanu.

Hair

Best carrier oils for hair include black seed, apricot kernel, jojoba, sesame seed, coconut, and sweet almond.

Joints

Best carrier oils for joints include emu, olive, borage, flaxseed, and jojoba.

Massage

Best carrier oils for massage include macadamia nut, sweet almond, sunflower, and jojoba.

Scar Healing

Best carrier oils for scar healing include neem, grape seed, rose hip, tamanu, and cocoa butter.

Skin

Best carrier oils for skin include black seed, avocado, carrot seed, rose hip, wheat germ, hemp seed, grape seed, jojoba, pomegranate, safflower, sweet almond, tamanu, and wheat germ.

Wound Healing

Best carrier oils for wounds and healing include apricot kernel, evening primrose, carrot seed, emu, avocado, and black seed.

Mixing Your Carrier and Essential Oils

When you want to make a remedy with essential oils, I suggest you start backward. Decide which carrier oil you want to use based on your end goal or product. If you want to make a light, smooth massage oil, use macadamia nut or sunflower carrier oil with your essential oil mix. If you want to make an antiaging skin cream, use wheat germ, pomegranate, argan, neem, or tamanu.

Pick what you want to accomplish and then choose the carrier oil and the essential oils that contain the properties for the issue you want to solve. Work from the goal backward. Combine them and you'll have double the power for effectiveness.

I mentioned shea butter and cocoa butter in the above lists. When mixed with essential oils, butters like shea and cocoa permit the essential oils to evaporate less quickly than carrier oils do. The essential oil can remain on the skin longer, which is good for certain applications like face creams and wound healing. The butters—shea, cocoa, mango, and kombo—spread the essential oils out for more even skin absorption, as well as protecting them from fast (volatile) evaporation. Therefore, the skin stays moister longer.

Dispersants

There is nothing like a warm, relaxing bath to take away your chills, anxieties, worries, stresses, exhaustion, aches and pains, sore muscles, sadness, or tightness. You can choose from many different essential oils to relieve your headaches, stress, or strain and add them to your bath. As you learn more about essential oils, you'll make a list of your favorites. But here are a few tips for the wise.

Just like using carrier oils to dilute your essential oils, you'll always need to dilute your essential oils when you add them to your bathwater. Be sure to dilute them, otherwise the essential oil will float to the top of the water and, at some point, encounter your tender skin. "Yeowie" is a familiar word heard from bathtubs around the world when essential oils are not first diluted and come into contact with human skin as an oily glob. Diluting allows your essential oils to disperse correctly in the bathwater. Here are the options:

Solubol

Mix one-part essential oil to eight parts Solubol, then add to bath.

Polysorbate 20 or Polysorbate 80

Mix five to twenty drops of essential oil with equal amounts of Polysorbate 20 or 80, then add to bath.

Natrasorb

This is a modified tapioca starch. Mix five to twenty drops of essential oil to two tablespoons of Natrasorb, then add to bath.

Castile Soap

Use five to twenty drops of essential oil per one tablespoon of castile soap, mix, and add to bath.

Vodka

Use 160–190 proof *only*. Mix five to twenty drops of essential oil in two tablespoons of vodka and add to bath. Never use less than 160 proof or the molecules will separate. Everclear is a grain alcohol brewed at a very high alcohol content.

Shampoo

Take ½ ounce of shampoo out of your bottle and mix with five to twenty drops of chosen essential oil. Use and repeat each time. Never pre-mix shampoo and essential oils and leave in the bottle. Always mix fresh each time. It is advisable to use a shampoo that is toxin free when using essential oils.

By taking care to dilute and correctly disperse essential oils, you will have a long and healthy relationship with your essential oil creating and products. It's so much better to be on the safe side of these amazing oils.

As you work more and more with carrier oils, you will discover the special ones that are your favorite go-to oils. The more I experiment with different carrier oils, the more respect I have for them. I can make the same product with two different carrier oils and it will turn out differently. I love the nut oils for face creams and lotions and I enjoy the seed oils for skin applications. You'll have your own favorites in no time, and you'll know which ones work best for the purpose you have chosen. Let's move on to the essential oils that have been selected as your introduction into the world of aromatherapy.

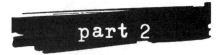

part 2

Twenty Essential Oils
to Start You Out

Welcome to the section on essential oils that covers twenty essential oils, in alphabetical order for your convenience. I know there's a lot of information to take in, but one of the things I encourage my beginning students to do is to familiarize themselves with the descriptions of each oil. Our brain only absorbs about 30 percent of the information in the first go-around, so if you read about the essential oil a few times, you'd have a thorough understanding of what they are and how they perform.

It's like getting to know a new friend. They might have to tell you their names and stories a few times before you remember them! No worries, though. It will happen. The more you chat with them and trade stories, the more you get to know them. Just don't be afraid to revisit and refresh these chapters so you have a working knowledge of each essential oil. I think it's like seeing a movie again; it becomes richer and deeper the second time around.

Each essential oil in this section will cover the basic information about that oil, its properties, its benefits, how it is obtained, some background and history of the essential oil, the creative uses for it, and the other oils it blends nicely with. Each description should give you a good overview of the oil and how it might be able to enhance your life. Starting in alphabetical order, we begin with bergamot.

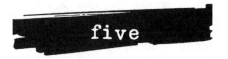

five

Bergamot *(Citrus bergamia)* Essential Oil

B ergamot is a small plant that produces a type of citrus fruit. Oil crushed from the peel of the fruit is used to make the essential oil. It's claimed that Arab traders brought it from China. The very savvy English used bergamot to flavor their Earl Grey tea blend. Bergamot essential oil was a very valuable commodity during the fifteenth and sixteenth centuries.

Originally, bergamot was named for an Italian city, *Bergamot*, where the essential oil was originally grown and sold. The Italians have used bergamot in natural medicine for years, in particular for fevers. The fruit was native to Southeast Asia and imported to the south of Italy, in the Calabria region. Now bergamot is extensively cultivated and grown in Argentina, Tunisia, Ivory Coast, Algeria, and Morocco.

Bergamot is most probably a hybrid of lemon and bitter orange. The oil is obtained from the cold expression of the peel of nearly ripe fruit of the bergamot tree. The small fruit tree produces round, very bitter, inedible (raw) fruit that resembles a miniature orange. Bergamot essential oil has a citrus-like aroma with a spicy undertone.

Bergamot is one of my favorite essential oils. I use it for sleep and as a mood enhancer when I need brightening. It's beautiful during the holidays, too.

Source

Bergamot essential oil is a cold-pressed oil obtained from the inside rind of the bergamot orange fruit. It smells slightly like an orange with a floral note and a sweetness to its smell.

Benefits

Bergamot essential oil is analgesic, antibiotic, stimulant, diuretic, antiseptic, antidepressant, deodorant, and sedative. It has been known to relieve urinary tract infections; boost liver functions; help balance the spleen and stomach; assist in reducing oily skin; curtail acne; clear up psoriasis, eczema, and cold sores; relieve depression; and alleviate tension and fear.

Italian research has shown that bergamot essential oil has a wide variety of medicinal uses as well as in culinary dishes. (I do not recommend you cook with it.) It also has superb antiseptic qualities that are useful for skin complaints such as acne, oily skin, eczema, and psoriasis, and can be used on cold sores, chicken pox, and wounds.

Bergamot essential oil is also helpful for respiratory problems, and mouth and urinary tract infections. For emotional disorders, it has helped with SAD (Seasonal Affective Disorder); and when one is feeling a bit off, lacking in self-confidence, reticent, or shy, bergamot essential oil can be diffused or inhaled for relief. Bergamot oil can also be used to treat depression, stress, tension, fear, hysteria, infection (all types, including skin), anorexia, psoriasis, eczema, and for general convalescence.

Precautions

Bergamot essential oil is highly phototoxic and should only be stored in dark bottles in cool, dark places to protect it from sunlight because it can become toxic if exposed to sunlight. Stay out of the sun for at least eight to twelve hours after it is diluted and applied or rubbed onto the skin.

Do not use bergamot essential oil in cases of severe liver problems. Check with your doctor if you are taking medications for liver disease. Do not use when pregnant or nursing. Bergamot essential oil can be a possible skin irritant. Discontinue use at least two weeks prior to surgery. Patch test a small area for sensitivity and always be sure to dilute well.

Creative Ways to Use Bergamot (Citrus bergamia) Essential Oil

- To reduce anxiety, inhale or diffuse a few drops of bergamot essential oil.

- Lift a dark mood, reduce anxiety, jittery nerves, nervous tension and stress by diffusing bergamot essential oil.

- Use as a spray to promote sleep. Mix ten drops of bergamot oil in one ounce of water. Shake well to mix the oil. Spray onto your pillow before bed to induce sleep.

- Inhaled or diffused, a few drops of bergamot essential oil can refresh the senses, improve mental alertness, balance the nervous system, fight infections, and promote faster illness recovery.

- Used in a diffuser, bergamot essential oil can help a person overcome a smoking habit by diverting the impulse to smoke and by regulating the appetite.

- A combination of bergamot and lavender essential oils mixed together can help with feelings of loss or grief by diffusing and inhaling the uplifting mist.

- To cool a fever, use ten drops properly dispersed (chapter 4) in a bath to help reduce the temperature.

- Bergamot essential oil can help to regulate the appetite when three to four drops are diffused.

- For a holiday treat, sprinkle a few drops of bergamot, myrrh, frankincense, or cinnamon bark essential oils on your holiday decorations to give them a festive scent.

- For a super uplifting bath, mix bergamot essential oil with any of these oils: clary sage, geranium, Melissa, or frankincense. Use one or two oils, mixed and dispersed, ten to fifteen drops total. (See chapter 4 for correct dispersants.)

Bergamot *(Citrus bergamia)* Essential Oil Blends Nicely With

Clary sage, frankincense, rose geranium, sandalwood, orange, rosemary, and ylang-ylang essential oils. It is particularly complementary with other citrus oils, too.

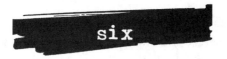

six

Clary Sage *(Salvia sclarea)* Essential Oil

M y oh my, what an interesting name you have, dear clary sage essential oil! The English named it clary, which originates in the Latin *sclarea*, a word derived from *clarus* (clear). Over time, this name was gradually modified to one of the more popular names, clear eye, since the seeds have been thought to be beneficial for clearing impaired sight. In olden times, the seeds were found to be mucilaginous, and a decoction made from them was placed in the affected eye to clear away small foreign bodies that might cause irritation. But don't be fooled by the name or the old use; this essential oil is *not* to be used in your eyes. There are horror stories about permanent corneal damage from drops put into delicate eyes. Be charmed by the name, but not enticed to use it incorrectly.

Clary sage is commonly known as *the gentler essential oil*. In certain parts of the world, specialty wine was made from the flowers of the herb. Combined with boiled sugar, it had a flavor like *Frontignac*, a sweet wine grape drink similar to Muscat. The smell is very herbal and earthy and has a floral and nutty tone. It smells like something directly from Mother Earth and, in that way, is a very comforting aroma.

Clary sage essential oil has been a powerful potion for centuries. It is particularly helpful in the management of pain. It is especially effective for the pain that can come from interior swelling, hormonal issues, childbirth, headaches, stomach inflammation, gall bladder irritation, and anything in the body that becomes inflamed.

Herbalists and midwives in many regions of the world have traditionally used clary sage essential oil to ease the painful tightening of the uterus during childbirth. Clary sage essential oil is frequently combined with geranium essential oil to facilitate controlling as well as alleviating disorders endured by women from hormonal imbalances like menopausal symptoms, irregular menstrual periods, depression, headache, and nausea. For relief of feminine symptoms, use a cool towel compress of diluted clary sage essential oil. The use of a similar compress, but warmed, alleviates liver, stomach, and gall bladder problems.

Clary sage essential oil is used to calm the nervous system, especially during times of trauma and stress, depression, and insomnia. It can provide anxiety-lifting effects.

Men, women, and children can all suffer from imbalances and inflammation from time to time, especially people undergoing treatment for cancer and those with inflammatory diseases. Clary sage essential oil is used to relieve pain as a compress and as a massage oil diluted in a carrier oil when and if the skin and area can be touched. If the area is too tender for hands, then use a heated or cooled compress and place gently on the area affected.

You can use a clary sage essential oil compress as a headache reliever when your headache originates from inflammation, like sinus irritation, or if you have overworked your muscles during exercise.

Source

Clary sage oil is extracted by distillation of the stems and leaves and flowering tips of the *Salvia sclarea* plant.

Benefits

Clary sage is antiseptic, antidepressant, anticonvulsive, antispasmodic, digestive, euphoric, (calming) nervine, sedative, stomachic, and uterine. Clary sage essential oil is used to enhance the immune system, calm digestive disorders, reduce inflammation from eczema, calm muscle spasms, and relieve respiratory ailments. It can help menstrual issues (cramps and hot flashes), promote relaxation during childbirth, and ease menopause symptoms.

Precautions

Do not use clary sage essential oil during the first trimester of pregnancy. And do not use if you are consuming alcohol, as it can cause hyper-intoxication. Clary sage essential oil is generally a safe and non-toxic essential oil, but may have some possibilities of irritating mucous membranes. Inhale clary sage essential oil carefully and in small amounts to prevent excessive states of euphoria.

Special Note: don't confuse clary sage essential oil with salvia officinalis or common sage essential oil, which is not recommended due to the high content of thujone (a toxic substance). Just because they both have sage in their name doesn't make them the same. *Salvia lavandulifolia* or Spanish sage essential oil, has many uses in aromatherapy but is not likely to offer the same benefits as clary sage essential oil. They come from the same genus but have very different properties and safety concerns.

Creative Ways to Use Clary Sage (*Salvia sclarea*) Essential Oil

- To break up mucus in the lungs, use one to three drops of clary sage essential oil in a diffuser.
- For relief of rheumatic pain and inflammation, mix three drops of clary sage essential oil with one drop of frankincense essential oil, one drop of eucalyptus essential oil, and one drop of rosemary essential oil to one tablespoon of carrier oil and massage onto inflamed or painful areas or joints.

- For general pain relief, mix two drops of clary sage essential oil with two drops of peppermint essential oil, three drops of lavender essential oil, and one tablespoon of carrier oil. Rub onto the affected areas. Diffuse the recipe (minus the carrier oil) when you need to see the big picture and get away from the minutia of the day.

- For a pick-me-up, mix seven drops of clary sage essential oil with ten drops of frankincense essential oil and eight drops of orange essential oil. Diffuse or mix with a carrier oil for a massage.

- For emotional support, mix one drop of clary sage essential oil with one drop each of sandalwood and lemon essential oils before diffusing.

- Reward and refresh yourself by inhaling or diffusing one drop each of clary sage, lavender, and marjoram essential oils.

- To control hot flashes, diffuse one drop of clary sage essential oil with one drop of basil, one drop of lavender, and one drop of rose essential oils.

- For help with hair loss, add a few drops of clary sage essential oil to your shampoo to stimulate hair growth. Clary sage essential oil can also be effective in alleviating dandruff.

- Clary sage essential oil can be used to cleanse wounds and may help protect the body during surgery and against infections. Mix three drops of clary sage essential oil to one teaspoon of antiseptic carrier oil. Apply carefully.

- Relieve headaches by diffusing three drops of clary sage essential oil. It can also be used for back pain, muscle stiffness, and cramps.

Clary Sage *(Salvia sclarea)* Essential Oil Blends Nicely With

Bergamot, frankincense, geranium, lavender, sandalwood, and pine essential oils.

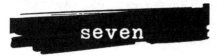

seven

Clove *(Syzygium aromaticum)* Essential Oil

C love bud essential oil is among the most powerful of all the aromatherapy oils. Native to the Indonesian Maluku Islands, cloves were a treasured commodity prized by the ancient Romans. This spice was among the first to be traded.

The Chinese also used cloves as early as 226 BCE. So the Emperor would not have bad breath in his royal presence, any visitor was commanded to masticate the *flowerettes* as a precaution against foul mouth odor. Physical evidence of cloves has been found in vessels dating as far back as 1721 BCE.

Cloves, and clove products, were one of the most precious spices of the sixteenth and seventeenth century. In 1605, the Dutch traders attempted to overtake and monopolize the clove trade. To corner the market, they sent ships and ill-intended crews to destroy clove trees that sprouted up anywhere outside of their control. The sad result was the citizens of Ternate, Maluku, had been epidemic-free until the Dutch ravaged their clove trees. Unprotected, thousands died from contagious diseases because they no longer had cloves to protect and naturally immunize them.

Due to the competition-crushing destructive actions of the Dutch, cloves were grown in other places in the eighteenth century, including Zanzibar, Madagascar, Brazil, Mauritius, Tidore, and Tanzania. The new supply allowed the prices to fall, and cloves became affordable to all classes of people.

This spice gets its name from the French word *clou*, which means nail. The clove bud is actually a dried flower bud that grows on the branches of an evergreen tree. It resembles a small nail when dried.

I always thought clove bud, or clove, was just a spice you use in holiday cookies and gingerbread. Once I began to explore the uses of clove essential oil, it opened new horizons for me. It helps me after a particularly strenuous yoga class when I have a few sore muscles. It helps with dental pain, and used in my diffuser, it keeps the house smelling great, even in the stuffy winter months. I take along a little clove essential oil to freshen up and purify the air of hotel rooms, too. It's a warm and tingly essential oil, and I like to have it close by for all kinds of practical reasons and emergencies.

Source

Clove essential oil is obtained by extracting the oil from the buds of the clove tree. It gives off a spicy, sweet, warm aroma that is pungent and strong.

Benefits

Clove bud essential oil is analgesic, antiseptic, antispasmodic, anti-infectious, disinfectant, insecticide, stimulant, and stomachic.

It can be used for acne, bruises, burns and cuts, keeping infections at bay, and as a pain reliever. It helps with toothaches, mouth sores, rheumatism, and arthritis.

It is beneficial to the digestive system, and is effective against vomiting, diarrhea, flatulence, spasms, and parasites, as well as bad breath. Clove bud essential oil relieves respiratory problems like bronchitis, asthma, and tuberculosis.

Due to its antiseptic properties, clove bud essential oil is useful for wounds, cuts, scabies, athlete's foot, fungal infections, bruises, prickly heat, scabies, and other types of injuries. It also has properties to repel moths and red fire ants.

Clove bud essential oil has long been used to aid in dentistry due to its anesthetic properties.

Precautions

Do not use while pregnant or if you have a liver or kidney condition. Clove bud essential oil may interact with certain drugs. Check with your physician before using. Clove bud essential oil is very strong and should always be used in diluted form. Avoid using on children under the age of two. Do a patch test on your skin before applying this powerful essential oil, as it may cause skin irritation. Tisserand and Young recommend a dermal maximum of .5 percent (Young, *Essential Oils Safety*, second edition, 2014).

Creative Ways to Use Clove (*Syzygium aromaticum*) Essential Oil

- For digestive problems: diffuse four to five drops of clove bud essential oil near the dining room before and after meals. Or dilute five drops of clove bud essential oil with one tablespoon of carrier oil and massage clockwise around abdominal region.

- For a room disinfectant: diffuse four drops of clove bud essential oil to kill germs and purify the air.

- Muscle aches and joint relief: mix eight drops of clove bud essential oil into two ounces of carrier oil (jojoba, borage, rose hip) and massage onto the affected area.

- For toothache: add a couple drops of diluted clove bud essential oil to a cotton swab and rub onto achy tooth for instant relief. This helps kill the infection-causing bacteria and reduces pain.

- For throat pain: mix one to two drops of clove bud essential oil to one cup of water. Gargle to reduce pain. Do not swallow.

- Bad breath help: mix one to two drops of clove bud essential oil to one cup of water. Gargle to clean mouth. Do not swallow.

- Stress relief: diffuse four to five drops of clove bud essential oil or inhale over steam with your eyes closed for a stimulating effect on the mind and to remove mental exhaustion and fatigue.

- For respiratory problems (coughs, colds, bronchitis, asthma, sinusitis): diffuse five drops of clove bud essential oil to curb the inflammation.

- Moths be gone: place a few drops of clove bud essential oil on some cotton balls. Put the cotton balls in your closet, drawers, and linen cabinet. Not only will the fragrance spice up your closet, it will also help to send moths away. Be sure your children or pets cannot access these balls. Place them in a small mesh bag for safety.

- For insect protection: combine five drops of clove bud essential oil with five drops of peppermint essential oil and two drops of lemon essential oil in a quart of water. Stir well. Pour the mixture into a spray bottle. Shake vigorously. Spritz the area around baseboards, under cabinets and appliances, and on countertops to repel common household pests. Reapply the mixture frequently in the summer months (once a week) and twice monthly in the winter. Be sure your pets cannot lick the mixture or toddlers can access the sprayed area.

Clove *(Syzygium aromaticum)* Essential Oil Blends Nicely With

Bergamot, chamomile, clary sage, cedarwood, geranium, ginger, grapefruit, lavender, lemon, rose, sandalwood, and ylang-ylang essential oils.

eight

Eucalyptus *(Eucalyptus globulus. E radiata)* Essential Oil

E ucalyptus essential oil is used as a fragrance in perfumes and cosmetics. It is found in toothpastes, mouthwashes, cough drops, ointments, and lozenges. Frequently, it is mixed with other oils to make it more easily absorbed by the skin.

Although similar in properties to tea tree essential oil, eucalyptus essential oil is a bit more effective for treating bronchial and respiratory infections, while tea tree essential oil is better as a topical antiseptic application due to its skin-friendly qualities. Owning both essential oils covers all your bases.

Australian aboriginals have used oil-containing eucalyptus leaf infusions as a traditional medication for body pains, fever, sinus congestions, and colds for centuries. It is favored by the natives as a general cure-all.

There are several different ways to use eucalyptus essential oil, including aromatically, topically, or by inhalation. For instance, it can be applied to skin diluted in a carrier oil, such as safflower, jojoba, or sweet almond oil. Start with two drops added to one to three teaspoons of carrier oil. Increase the eucalyptus essential oil as needed, but don't exceed the recommended amount in the dilution chart for safety.

There are more than 500 different species of Eucalyptus (Eucalypts) grown and cultivated. Because of the wide variety, it is important to know which species of this essential oil you purchase. Below is a description of the four most popular ones:

Eucalyptus globulus: best known and most used for eucalyptus essential oils.

Eucalyptus radiata: commonly known as the narrow-leaved peppermint tree.

These two are used to ease congestion and sinus pressure due to colds, flu, and bronchitis. Mixed with a carrier oil, they are perfect for easing muscle aches and arthritis pain. Mixed with a carrier oil, they can repel insects and can ease the sting and pain of insect bites.

There are two other versions that are used, but not as common as the first two.

Eucalyptus citriodora: called the lemon-scented gum, the principal constituent of the oil is citronellal, used for industrial and perfume purposes. Many outdoor candles feature this oil as a mosquito repellant. However, the effects of this oil diffused only lasts about one hour.

Eucalyptus polybractea: called the Blue mallee, or Blue-leaved mallee tree. This version is best used in the laundry as a washing agent, to clean the floors, and as a household antiseptic. It can purify the air when diffused.

Eucalypts (the official name for the tree) were first seen by early European explorers to Australia. However, no botanical collections are known to have been made until 1777 when botanist David Nelson collected a eucalypt on Bruny Island, southern Tasmania, and took it back to England. There are also products from French-grown eucalypts, but this book recommends the ones grown in Australia for the truest source of your essential oils.

In 1948, the United States also officially registered eucalyptus oil as an insecticide and miticide (kills mites and ticks).

My mother emigrated from Australia after WWII to marry my father. We made several trips to Australia when I was growing up and I was very familiar with the day-to-day household use of eucalyptus essential oil and tea tree oil. You could say these were not only the insect repellants for the tropical climates of Brisbane and Sydney, but also the household cleaners of choice for my Australian grandmother and aunts. They used a bucket (no spray bottles back then) filled with water, white vinegar, and eucalyptus essential oil to clean the kitchen floors, counters, sideboards, and tables. They used this formula for the bathrooms: two cups of water, one cup of white vinegar, and twenty to thirty drops of eucalyptus polybractea (Blue mallee) essential oil to get the job done.

If we were headed to the park for a picnic, Granny would whip up mosquito repellant in a glass bottle and apply it to my arms, face, and legs. She would have to do this once an hour, but it kept my arms from looking like a buffet dinner for the hungry mosquitoes.

Source

The leaves of the eucalyptus tree are steam distilled to produce the oil high in 1,8-cineole and α-pinene. It has been described as smelling like minty pine with a touch of honey.

Benefits

Having powerful antimicrobial, antiviral, antibacterial, and antifungal properties, eucalyptus essential oil has been effectively used as an expectorant, for respiratory blockages, sinus infections, asthma, bronchitis, inflammation, coughs, and as an antiseptic and treatment option for wounds, burns, and ulcers.

As early as the 1880s, surgeons were already using eucalyptus essential oil for antiseptic cleansing during operations. Eucalyptus oil has also been used as an insect repellant and often in combination with other essential oils.

Precautions

Eucalyptus essential oil is strong and should not be used on babies or children under two years, even diluted. It has been known to cause respiratory problems in young children. The maximum concentration when mixed with a carrier oil should be 20 percent. (To achieve this ratio, mix twenty drops of eucalyptus essential oil to one tablespoon of carrier oil for short term use only.)

Creative Ways to Use Eucalyptus (*Eucalyptus globulus. E radiata*) Essential Oil

- Apply a drop of eucalyptus essential oil to a cotton ball and sniff it several times a day to heal mucus membranes and to treat allergies or asthma.
- Add a few drops of eucalyptus essential oil to water or a nebulizer as a steam therapy for coughs, colds, or sinus inflammation and chest congestion. Add four drops of frankincense essential oil if the cough has settled.
- Steam out a cold with five drops each of eucalyptus, thyme, tea tree, and lavender essential oils.
- To decongest and heal a respiratory infection, diffuse four drops of eucalyptus essential oil for twenty to thirty minutes three times a day. Halve the time for children under twelve.
- Apply diluted eucalyptus essential oil to the soles of your feet to help with a cold, cough, or congestion. (Five drops of eucalyptus essential oil to one teaspoon of carrier oil.)
- Put a drop or two of diluted eucalyptus essential oil on a blister to alleviate the swelling and to disinfect the area.
- Try eucalyptus essential oil, diluted and dispersed, in a sponge bath to reduce fevers.

- Create an antiviral spray: mix ten drops of eucalyptus essential oil with ten drops of tea tree essential oil, four drops of thyme essential oil, and six drops of lavender essential oil in ten ounces of clean water and use as an air spray for the home or office. Shake well before spraying.

- Use as an effective antiseptic on herpes and shingles. Modify your dilution beginning with two to three drops per teaspoon and make sure your carrier oil is 100 percent pure.

- Use a few drops of eucalyptus essential oil to speed up the healing of wounds and skin ulcers. Add a few drops to an antiseptic or therapeutic cream or lotion for pain relief.

- Use diluted eucalyptus essential oil on your skin for relief of insect bites or wounds but be very careful when doing so. Use only a drop at a time.

- Use as a wash to cleanse wounds. Mix a few drops in clean, warm water and use a sterile cloth on wounds.

- Add ten drops of eucalyptus essential oil per one ounce of shampoo to help maintain beautiful hair and a healthy scalp.

- To disinfect surfaces, add ten to twenty drops of eucalyptus essential oil to a spray bottle and add warm water. (You can also add a few drops of lemon essential oil if you like.) Using this eucalyptus essential oil spray on bedding and mattresses can help eliminate bed bugs.

- Add eucalyptus essential oil to your detergent when you wash your sheets to help eliminate bed bugs and dust mites. (You can also freeze your sheets to kill those pesky mites.)

Eucalyptus *(Eucalyptus globulus. E radiata)* Essential Oil Blends Nicely With

Tea tree, lavender, thyme, Melissa, lemon, basil, bergamot, orange, peppermint, and rosemary essential oils.

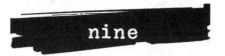
Frankincense *(Boswellia carterii)* Essential Oil

C ommonly known as frankincense to westerners, the resin is called *olibanum*, and in Arabic *al-lubān*. The definition is based on a visual of how the resin is grown and harvested: *that which results from milking or the product resulting from the sap of the Boswellia tree.* Like many other herbs, essential oils, and spices, frankincense was brought to Europe by the Crusaders.

Frankincense *(boswellia carteri)* comes from the boswellia genus trees, particularly *boswellia sacra* and *boswellia carteri.* When the milky white sap is extracted from the tree bark, it is hardened for several days into a gum resin and then scraped off in perfect tear-shaped droplets. Originally only the King's merchants were allowed to harvest and use frankincense because the ruler owned all the trees. Hence, frankincense was considered sacred and hard to acquire for common folk.

The English word frankincense came from an old French term, *franc encens,* which translates to *high quality incense.* In ancient French, the meaning for the word *franc* was *noble or pure.* No wonder that became a popular name and description of the essential oil because it has so many amazing qualities.

Frankincense is traditionally burned as incense and was charred and ground into a powder to produce the heavy kohl eyeliner used by ancient makeup artists. It was applied to upper-class Egyptian women and royalty (like the classic artwork and Hollywood movies portray).

When the resin is steam-distilled, it produces an aromatic essential oil with a bounty of benefits. In ancient Egypt, frankincense was revered as the *sweat of the gods.*

Recent studies have indicated that the worldwide frankincense tree populations are declining due partly to overexploitation and the ravages of the longhorn beetle. Only responsible farmers who are conscientious about preservation and use sustainable methods for growing and harvesting will keep this sacred tree alive for generations to come. As a rule, when using natural products, we should only patronize those growers and manufacturers who practice sustainability so subsequent generations can enjoy the benefits of this wonderful, natural substance. Try to ensure you are buying from these sources.

I grew up attending church services where the priest carried a *thurible* up the center aisle to infuse the church with smoking frankincense. The first time I burned frankincense in my home, it took me back to hard pews and strict nuns.

I eventually became quite fond of the healing aroma of the actual incense. Now, I prefer to obtain all the healing benefits of the oil without the ceremony and smoke.

Source

Frankincense oil is steam distilled from the resin of the Boswellia tree. The aroma is resinous and earthy, with a slightly fruity/sweet, warm, spicy scent to it.

Benefits

Frankincense is known for its anti-inflammatory, astringent, tonic, antiseptic, disinfectant, digestive, diuretic, expectorant, uterine, and vulnerary (wound healing) properties.

Frankincense has been very effective in helping a number of complaints in the body. It can aid the absorption of nutrients and strengthen the immune system. Frankincense essential oil has been found useful for certain health conditions like rheumatoid arthritis, stomach ulcers, asthma, breaking up phlegm, and helping digestive disorders by stimulating gastric juices and bile production.

The antiseptic qualities of this oil can help prevent bad breath, cavities, toothaches, mouth sores, and other infections. Frankincense essential oil often regulates estrogen production in women and reduces the risk of post-menopausal tumor or cyst formation in the uterus (uterine cancer). It also can regulate the menstrual cycle of premenopausal women.

Frankincense essential oil is studied globally for its potential to treat cancer. Scientists have observed that there is an agent in this oil that not only stops cancer from spreading, but also induces cancerous cells to close themselves down. Immunologist Mahmoud Suhail is hoping to open a new chapter in the history of frankincense.[3]

Precautions

Frankincense essential oil should not be used during pregnancy. Avoid using if the oil has oxidized. You can tell if the oil is cloudy, smells off, or has become thick and viscous.

Creative Ways to Use Frankincense
(Boswellia carteri) Essential Oil

- Use as a wrinkle relief (night or day) cream by adding a few drops of frankincense essential oil to the base cream or lotion of your choice.

- Place a few drops of frankincense essential oil on your washcloth and run it over yourself during your final shower (warm) rinse. The steam will infuse the frankincense essential oil and you get the benefit of a quick and refreshing *frankincensed* steam bath.

- If you want to enjoy a special indulgence, use frankincense essential oil in the bath with a proper dispersant. (This breaks up the oil and spreads it out in the water.)

- Treat dry skin by mixing a few drops of frankincense essential oil in a teaspoon of carrier oil, like sweet almond, pomegranate, kukui nut, tamanu, argan, or carrot oil and massage it onto your face.

3. Howell, Jeremy. *BBC World News*. February 9. (Accessed December 15, 2018.) http://news.bbc.co.uk/2/hi/middle_east/8505251.stm.

- Treat wrinkles and the signs of aging by adding two drops of frankincense essential oil to your nightly moisturizing cream or lotion treatment. Add one to two drops of sandalwood essential oil for an even richer treatment.

- Reduce the appearance of stretch marks and scars by mixing two drops of frankincense essential oil with two drops of lavender essential oil and one drop of helichrysum essential oil in one tablespoon of carrier oil. Massage onto scar tissue.

- For a revitalizing face serum, mix two drops of frankincense essential oil and two drops of lavender essential oil in one ounce of carrier oil. Massage onto skin using an upward motion.

- Diffuse or inhale a few drops of frankincense essential oil directly to lift your mood.

- To strengthen hair roots, mix a few drops of frankincense essential oil with double the drops of a carrier oil like jojoba, coconut, or sesame seed.

- Speed up the healing of cuts, acne, insect bites, and boils using diluted frankincense essential oil. Perform a patch test for safety and use a small drop of diluted frankincense essential oil on acne or a bite.

Frankincense *(Boswellia carteri)* Essential Oil Blends Nicely With

Lemon, orange, bergamot, lavender, sandalwood, other citrus oils, rose geranium, and Melissa essential oils.

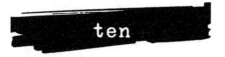

ten

Lavender *(Lavandula angustifolia)* Essential Oil

The first essential oil I always recommend is lavender *(lavendula angustofolia)*. If you could have only one essential oil, I believe it should be lavender. It is one of the gentlest of all the essential oils and yet is one of the most versatile, and is therefore my first choice. It's like the question: "If you could only take one book with you to a desert island, what would it be?" Only this time, the question is about an essential oil. I would unequivocally take lavender.

Ancient records describing lavender plants have been found in Greece, where the purple flower got its name from the Syrian city of Naarda. Lavender was originally called nardus. The Greeks loved lavender and passed it on to the Romans who used it to wash their clothes, linens, and perfume their famous communal baths.

The famous floral fragrance has been used by many cultures for centuries because it has therapeutically calming, relaxing, and balancing properties that register both physically and emotionally. Lavender has been used as a perfume, in cooking, as an aid for depression, as an immune system builder, and has shown it can relieve anxiety and fatigue. It is also highly famous for its skin-healing properties.

Lavender essential oil was the very first essential oil I ever tried. It was in the 1980s and I worked very long hours in television production. Our schedules were brutal. We were on call at 7 a.m. and often worked on the set until nine or ten in the evening. The next day, we'd do it all over again, often seven days a week. When I finally got a chance to sleep, my nervous system was wound tight from the day and there was always nerve-based anticipation for the next day's work.

Someone recommended lavender essential oil and I bought a bottle. Its pleasant aroma easily sent me to sleep.

Source

Lavender essential oil is steam distilled from the leaves, flowers, and buds of the lavender plant. It has a mild, pleasant scent that is floral and sweet with a hint of herbal undertones.

Benefits

Lavender is most commonly known for its relaxing effects on the body and mind. Throughout the ages, it has been highly revered for healing because it possesses antimicrobial, antibacterial, antifungal, and anti-inflammatory properties and is a relaxant and a nervine.

These same properties do wonders for the hair and scalp. Lavender even works as a natural bug repellant when mixed with other essential oils. Lavender essential oil is a natural remedy for insomnia, motion sickness, stress, anxiety, fatigue, and headaches.

Research has found that exposing yourself to the scent of lavender reduces postoperative pain, childbirth pain, and menstrual cramps. That's because the scent of lavender increases alpha waves, which are slower than beta waves, which are the normal electrical activity of the brain when awake. The wave activity is in the back of the brain, and when the lavender scent reaches the posterior part of the brain, it triggers the relaxing effect. When people are more relaxed and less anxious, they are less susceptible to pain. An anxious person feels pain more intensely than a calm and relaxed person.

Precautions

Lavender essential oil is one of the safest essential oils you can use. Lavandin and lavender do not have the exact same chemistry. Lavandin is known as Dutch Lavender (*Lavandula x intermedia*) and has slightly more camphor in the chemical composition. A standard caution is not to use lavender for infants under the age of six months. Some physicians caution to not use lavender essential oil two weeks prior to surgery. There is a concern for bleeding and an incompatible mix with prescribed medicines or those used during surgical procedures. Possible skin sensitization can occur. Do not use this essential oil if you have estrogen-dependent cancer or before operating heavy machinery.

Creative Ways to Use Lavender
(*Lavandula angustifolia*) Essential Oil

- Soothe your minor skin burns with two to three drops of diluted lavender essential oil.
- Rub diluted lavender essential oil lip balm on sun-burned, dry, or chapped skin and lips to moisturize.
- Minimize scar tissue by using a dilution of lavender essential oil and a carrier oil, like rose hip or neem.
- A single drop of lavender essential oil diluted and applied to a minor cut can kill bacteria while also helping to stop the bleeding and heal the wound.
- A single drop diluted and applied will reduce the itching of a bee sting or a cold sore.
- Mix several drops of lavender essential oil with a pure carrier oil and use topically for skin conditions like eczema, psoriasis, and dermatitis.
- Diffuse a few drops of lavender essential oil to minimize the effects of hay fever, pollen, seasonal change, and air-quality discomforts.
- To repel bugs, mix fifteen drops of lavender essential oil and five drops of eucalyptus oil in two tablespoons of carrier oil and rub on your skin. Repeat every two hours.
- Alleviate the symptoms of motion sickness by placing a drop of diluted lavender essential oil behind your ears or around your navel.

- Apply a few drops of diluted lavender essential oil to your hands and rub on a child's pillow to assist them with sleep. (The child should be over six months old.)

- Diffuse lavender essential oil to set the mood for pleasant social gatherings. (Make sure no one is sensitized to lavender before diffusing into the common air.)

- Diffuse or inhale lavender essential oil at the end of the day to release tension and refresh your mind, body, and spirit.

- Rub two to three drops of diluted lavender essential oil in your cupped palms, then inhale the scent to establish calm, invoke sleep, or even relieve hay fever.

- Rub diluted lavender mixture on your feet, temples, and wrists (or anywhere except the genitals) to bring about an immediate calming effect.

- Minimize dandruff by massaging diluted lavender essential oil into your scalp. (Apricot kernel would be a good carrier oil choice.)

- Use diluted lavender essential oil in crowded areas like planes or subways to create your personal oasis. Use in hotel rooms to aid tranquility and help your body recover from jet lag.

- Create more restful sleep by inhaling a few drops of diluted lavender essential oil rubbed into the palms of your hands and then smoothed onto your pillow.

- Place a few drops of lavender essential oil on a wet cloth or add to a dryer sheet to deodorize and freshen your laundry.

- Repel moths and insects by adding a few drops of lavender essential oil to cotton balls before placing them in closets and drawers. (Be sure you guard them from curious pets and children. Place them in a small mesh bag to prevent access to the cotton balls.)

- Scent your linen drawer in the same way as above using a saturated cotton ball of lavender essential oil contained in a mesh bag for safety.

- Make sachets filled with cotton balls doused with lavender essential oil.

Lavender *(Lavandula angustifolia)* Essential Oil Blends Nicely With

Bergamot, Roman chamomile, clary sage, clove, eucalyptus, geranium, grapefruit, lemon, patchouli, peppermint, rose, rosemary, tea tree, and thyme essential oils.

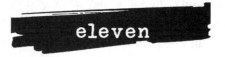
Lemon *(Citrus x limon)* Essential Oil

The earliest lemons originated in Asia. The curious yellow fruit was transported on ships by ancient explorers and merchants returning to Europe from East Asia. Their ships and camels were stacked high with fancy yarn goods and spices destined for Italy and the Mediterranean. They added bushels of this tasty yellow fruit to their cargo, which seemed to be as useful as a food as it was for a deck swab.

The earliest record of lemons in America suggested that they arrived on the ships with Christopher Columbus in 1493. Fresh lemons kept the sailors from getting scurvy on their long journey from Europe to the New World.

Lemons are extremely sensitive to cold temperatures and high humidity, therefore they grow best in the milder climates of southern California, Florida, and the Mediterranean region. They flourish in abundant, fragrant orchards in southern areas with ample sun.

Lemons are extensively used in kitchens and natural pharmacies. Many healers claim the lemon is an important healer and a staple for maintaining vibrant health. Lemons are invigorating, cleansing, uplifting, and inspiring. As such, we can use lemon essential oil for a variety of purposes ranging from medicinal, to health management, to cleaning, to purifying, and to keeping the air and environment germ free.

Besides the culinary benefits, I've used lemon juice to enhance the summer highlights in my hair. I know a few blondes who are blonder due to the power of the lemon. I characterize lemons as being a fun fruit with a multitude of applications, from diet and cleaning to beauty.

Lemon essential oil is wonderfully handy as an antiseptic and as an antibacterial cleaner for the kitchen and bathrooms. I also mix it with peppermint essential oil when I need a boost of energy. Combined, I inhale the oils and get the pick-me-up I need in the moment.

I always carry a little vial of aloe vera gel mixed with lemon and lavender essential oils drops. This is my portable hand sanitizer and it keeps my skin soft and germ free.

Source

Lemon essential oil comes from cold pressing lemon rinds. You will find some steam-distilled lemon and citrus oil on the market. Those are more for perfumes than therapeutic uses. Lemons have a clean, biting, sharp citrus fragrance.

Benefits

Lemon essential oil is astringent, antimicrobial, antibacterial, auto-immune supporting, a detoxifier, and antifungal. Stimulating and calming, lemon essential oil prevents infection; works at sleep inducing; acts as a digestive; can disperse cellulite; helps with varicose veins, anxiety, weight loss, and parasites; serves as a wrinkle wrangler; and is a refreshing addition to pretty much anything.

Precautions

Lemon essential oil is powerfully astringent and antiseptic. Any dilutions exceeding 5 percent should not be applied to skin because it can cause skin irritation in sensitive individuals. When you use any dilution of lemon essential oil directly on your skin, stay out of direct sunlight for at least eight to twelve hours and apply a sunscreen before venturing outdoors.

Creative Ways to Use Lemon (*Citrus x limon*) Essential Oil

- A few drops of diluted lemon essential oil rubbed on your chest and/or throat will help relieve congestion, coughs, and colds.
- Diffuse a few drops of lemon essential oil to alleviate any other respiratory complaints.
- Use well-diluted lemon essential oil (one drop) behind the ear or under the nose two to three times a day to

help fight seasonal allergies and hay fever. (Note: stay out of the sunlight if you apply topically.) Alternatively, you can apply diluted lemon essential oil to the bottoms of your feet using a rollerball you make yourself. (Be sure you patch test your skin for sensitivity.)

• Keep your toothbrush germ free by using one drop of lemon essential oil on your toothbrush and twirling it in a bit of water to sanitize. Rinse well.

• Four drops of lemon essential oil added to four ounces of warm water becomes a cleansing gargle for bad breath. It is also an effective mouthwash for mouth sores. Do not swallow.

• To treat acne, apply three drops of diluted lemon essential oil to a cotton ball and cleanse the affected area, repeating up to three times a day. Be careful of sun exposure after use on face. Wait eight to twelve hours.

• To achieve windows that shine without streaks, mix 50 percent water with 50 percent white vinegar and add ten to twenty drops of lemon essential oil into a spray bottle. Shake well before using. Spray and wipe clean with paper towels. (You may find that it takes a little more time for the surface to dry than with commercial cleaners, but you have the advantage of using a chemical- and alcohol-free cleaner, so you're not inhaling chemicals.)

• For a general disinfectant around the house, mix three drops of lemon essential oil with two ounces of water and shake vigorously before wiping down wooden furniture and kitchen chopping blocks. Use a stronger mixture as a kitchen board and counter sanitizer.

- For an energy pick-me-up, moisten a cloth with five drops of lemon essential oil and five drops of water. Hold the cloth directly underneath your nose and breathe in the scent for at least two to three minutes.

- For effective stress relief, add ten to fifteen drops of properly dispersed lemon essential oil to your bathwater and soak for at least fifteen minutes. Adding a few drops of lavender essential oil increases stress relief. Avoid sun exposure after your bath.

- For treating minor wounds, place five drops of lemon essential oil in a bowl of three ounces of clean warm water. Using a sterilized cloth dipped in the mixture, gently wipe the wound until it's clean.

- To eradicate nail fungus, apply two to three drops of diluted lemon essential oil to the nail in question several times a day. Note: have patience. It may take a few weeks or even months to fully clear up.

- For brighter skin and complexion, add a drop or two of lemon essential oil to your nighttime moisturizer. It's very important you don't do this in the morning since lemon oil (and most citrus oils) increase your sensitivity to the sun.

- For a clearer mind, diffuse a few drops of lemon essential oil in your office or study space to enhance mental clarity and concentration.

- Add a few drops of lemon essential oil plus two teaspoons of baking soda to your toilet to clean and sanitize the bowl.

- Rid yourself of more kitchen germs by soaking kitchen cloths and rags for twelve hours in a bowl of water containing two to three drops of lemon essential oil.

- Add eight drops to a diffuser and let the lemon essential oil clean and freshen the air.

- Add four to five drops of lemon essential oil to several cotton balls and place them into athletic shoes or a diaper pail for odor control. (Be sure pets and small children cannot access the soaked cotton balls.)

- Add a drop of lemon essential oil to the final rinse cycle on laundry day to make your laundry smell like fresh lemons.

- Lemon essential oil is an excellent grease remover. Dilute in a carrier oil and skin test before using on grime from your hands, as well as tools, dishes, and assorted household items. Wear gloves when using full strength.

- Lemon essential oil is a whiz at removing tree sap and the residue of glues from labels. Apply neat to objects or slightly diluted in a carrier oil.

- For oily or greasy hair, add three to four drops of lemon essential oil to wet hands, apply to freshly washed hair, then rinse. This treatment reduces the need for frequent shampooing and adds shine.

- To heal bug bites, apply two drops of diluted lemon essential oil directly to the bite and lightly rub. Repeat this process two times during the day. Remember, lemon essential oil increases photosensitivity. Be careful of the sun's ultraviolet rays.

Lemon *(Citrus x limon)*
Essential Oil Blends Nicely With

Lavender, rose, sandalwood, rose geranium, rosemary, ylang-ylang, and tea tree essential oils.

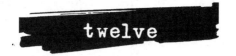

twelve

Melissa *(Melissa officinalis)* Essential Oil

M elissa essential oil *(Melissa officinalis)* is also commonly known as lemon balm and has many creative uses. The very name "Melissa" is Greek for "Honey Bee." *Melissa officinalis* was originally planted next to bee hives in order to encourage the production of a more delicious honey. Melissa essential oil is considered one of the most effective medicinal-oriented essential oils in aromatherapy and exudes a unique, herbaceous, pleasing and sweet scent.

According to Greek mythology, Melissa was a nymph who discovered and circulated the use of honey. It is believed she gave the bees their name.

True Melissa essential oil can be identified by its own unique aroma and properties. The cost is high because it takes 3.5 to 7.5 tons of plant material to produce one pound of essential oil. If Melissa essential oil is priced too low, it is likely to be adulterated in some way and will not contain the healing properties of the *true* Melissa essential oil.

Initially used as a culinary spice, Melissa lemon balm was easily grown as a windowsill herb and a type of vegetable. Famous and treasured for its limonene aroma and its mild flavor, Melissa was used as an alternative to mint and lemon in peasant cuisines. It is commonly added to soups, stews, salads, and a number of meat-based and seafood-based dishes.

The beauty of Melissa essential oil's gentle nature is that it can bring out those same qualities in people who use it. It is calming and at the same time uplifting, a source of relief for tension-induced headaches, and helps to balance the emotions. It encourages optimism and a sense of hope.

One of my favorite uses of Melissa essential oil is in salves and creams. It has such a light and heavenly smell that it somehow transports my mind to places like ancient Greece, Delphi, and the gleaming white marble columns. I seem to be able to tap into a higher realm whenever I use Melissa essential oil. Maybe it's because I like the story of its origin, but maybe there's something else going on too. I believe these plants were put on our earth to keep us connected not only to the earth, but to creation itself. As a result, many of the essential oils are happy to oblige and transport us to places beyond the plane of current reality, if we wish to go there with them. Melissa essential oil is one of those angelic messengers for me.

Source

Melissa essential oil is steam distilled from the leaves and flowers of the *Melissa officinalis* plant. It has a wonderfully fresh smell that presents a lemony and slightly herbaceous scent.

Benefits

Antidepressant, cordial (heart tonic), calming, sedative, antibacterial, and tonic, Melissa essential oil is used to help with symptoms of depression, colds and viruses, nervous disorders, PMS and menopause, hormonal issues, menstrual cramps, irregular periods, irritability, and depression. It has sedative and antispasmodic properties and has been used to help alleviate anxiety, anger, aggression, and irritability in those who suffer from Alzheimer's or dementia.

Melissa essential oils helps digestive system juices and warms the respiratory system. It is also the main ingredient in the famous Carmelite Water, created by medieval Carmelite nuns to treat nervousness and headaches. Carmelite Water was also known to enhance the complexion because of this main essential oil ingredient.

Melissa essential oil is highly regarded as a medicinal salve, because it can be used for infections and for minor to moderate skin injuries. It is also an analgesic as it brings pain relief to the injury.

Melissa is physically calming, uplifting, and soothing and produces a feeling of joyfulness and revitalization. Melissa essential oil is a top star in emotional and physical well-being. Melissa is one of those essential oils that must be experienced. It is complex, yet it is gentle. Its benefits, when applied correctly, will delight and astound you. It is a beautiful essential oil. I find it a wonderful fragrance for meditation and a deep, quiet massage. The scent enriches the moment for me and adds a level of serenity and happiness.

Precautions

Pregnant women should avoid this essential oil during the initial five months of pregnancy.

It's best to use Melissa essential oil in low concentrations. No more than a .9 percent dermal maximum and do not use in children and infants under age two and for those with hypersensitive/diseased/damaged skin.[4]

Dilute Melissa essential oil with appropriate carrier oils and/or by blending it with other essential oils or dispersants before using.

Creative Ways to Use Melissa
(Melissa officinalis) Essential Oil

- Reduce stress and anxiety by diffusing four drops of Melissa essential oil to fill the room with calm.
- For a mood enhancer, diffuse four drops of Melissa essential oil and two drops of lemon essential oil with one drop of bergamot essential oil to brighten your spirits.
- To comfort during times of grief and vulnerability, blend four drops Melissa essential oil with one drop frankincense essential oil in two teaspoons of a car-

---

4. Robert Tisserand and Rodney Young, *Essential Oils Safety second edition* (United Kingdom: Churchill Livingstone Elsevier, 2014), 351.

rier oil (like jojoba, apricot kernel, pomegranate, or tamanu) and use as a massage oil working clockwise around the upper torso.

- For headaches and migraines, add two drops Melissa essential oil to one teaspoon of jojoba, tamanu, or sweet almond oil and massage around forehead, temples, or neck.

- For restful sleep, diffuse four to five drops of Melissa essential oil and deeply inhale five times. You should experience calm.

- To ease the blues, diffuse three drops of Melissa essential oil with three drops of peppermint essential oil and three drops of bergamot essential oil. You can also add Melissa and bergamot essential oils to one tablespoon of carrier oil or lotion for massage.

- For anger or resentment relief, diffuse a blend of two drops of Melissa essential oil, one drop of bergamot essential oil, and one drop of lavender essential oil.

- For chronic fatigue or post-viral conditions, diffuse three drops of Melissa essential oil, three drops of black pepper essential oil, and five drops of orange essential oil.

- For a fatigue relief massage, blend five drops of rosemary essential oil, five drops of Melissa essential oil, five drops of neroli or basil essential oil, and one tablespoon of carrier oil. To use this in a bath, mix this blend with a proper dispersant and soak for fifteen minutes in the tub.

- To help with carpel tunnel syndrome, blend five drops of Melissa essential oil with five drops of lavender essential oil, one drop of clove bud essential oil, and one drop of black pepper essential oil. Add to a basin of warm water large enough to soak your hands and five inches above your wrists. Use a dispersant to distribute the essential oils. Soak for five to ten minutes.

- To use as a skin restoration cream, combine one half cup of shea butter and one tablespoon of borage oil with one teaspoon of honey and heat until they combine. When cooled, blend in twenty drops of Melissa essential oil, two drops of peppermint essential oil, and five drops each of helichrysum and sandalwood essential oils. Store in a sterilized dark glass jar and keep in a cool place. Apply twice daily.

Melissa *(Melissa officinalis)*
Essential Oil Blends Nicely With

Basil, Roman chamomile, lavender, rose geranium, rose, orange, lemon, bergamot, and ylang-ylang essential oils.

thirteen

Orange *(Citrus sinensis)*
Essential Oil

Orange essential oil is sunny, radiant, and brings happiness and warmth to the nose and mind along with a sense of cheerfulness and joy. It makes you want to dance! Historically, oranges have been associated with generosity and gratitude, and symbolized innocence and fertility. On Chinese New Year, oranges are given as gifts to symbolize happiness and prosperity.

In 1987, orange trees were designated as the most cultivated fruit tree in the world. Orange trees are widely grown in tropical and subtropical climates for their sweet fruit. Statistics from the Food and Agricultural Organization of the

United Nations 2013 show that sweet oranges accounted for approximately 70 percent of all citrus production worldwide.

Sweet oranges were mentioned in Chinese literature as far back as 314 BCE. How they got to Europe is uncertain, but we can logically assume trees or cuttings were transported via the busy Arab traders who brought goods and spices to the European continent in the eleventh century. Ships and camels were certainly most involved.

Orange fruit is a hybrid of pomelo *(citrus maxima)* and mandarin *(citrus reticulata)*. Genetically it is 25 percent pomelo and 75 percent mandarin. Orange essential oil is extracted from the orange peel by cold pressing.

Sweet orange essential oil is one of the most difficult oils to preserve. It has a shelf life of about six to twelve months, although if carefully stored in a cool area away from light, you may get more months of potency. Other citrus oils that have an orange-similar aroma are neroli, bergamot, mandarin, tangerine, petti grain, and yuzu.

One of the main reasons I wanted to move to California in the 70s was for the romantic experience of picking fresh oranges off the trees. So far, every orange tree I have ever planted has given beautiful fruit, but the backyard squirrels have systematically beaten me to the spoils of my gardening labors. Part of my current spiritual practice is centered around forgiving them and wishing them well. I buy my oranges at the farmers market and let the squirrels have the backyard bounty.

Source

Sweet orange essential oil is extracted by cold pressing the rinds of the orange. Orange essential oil gives off a sweet, fresh, perky, fruity scent. The blossoms smell super sweet to attract the pollinating bees.

Benefits

Sweet orange essential oil possesses qualities that are anti-inflammatory, antidepressant, antiseptic, aphrodisiac, diuretic, tonic, and sedative. Orange essential oil is used in aromatherapy to create the feelings of safety, happiness, and warmth, while calming nervous digestive problems. Sweet orange essential oil supplies cold and flu relief, rids the body of toxins, and stimulates the lymphatic system while assisting collagen formation in layers of the skin. It helps with insomnia, brightens a dull complexion, acts as a diuretic, reduces wrinkles, and has the amazing ability to foster sleep. Orange essential oil can be used effectively on the immune system, as well as for colds and flu and to eliminate toxins from the body.

Precautions

Orange essential oil is likely phototoxic and makes your skin sensitive to the sun. After you apply orange essential oil or a cream, lotion, or blend containing orange essential oil, it is advisable to wait eight to twelve hours before you go out in the sun. Tisserand and Young state that Bitter Orange essential oil is phototoxic, but cold pressed or steam distilled sweet orange is not.[5] However, it is a citrus, so I like to use caution and use an SPF 50 sunscreen or better for protection when I go out in the sun after use.

Creative Ways to Use Orange (*Citrus sinesis*) Essential Oil

- Use three to four drops of orange essential oil in a diffuser to help children and adults fall asleep and to alleviate the symptoms of cold and flu, nervous tension, and stress. Do not leave children unattended with the diffuser for more than a few minutes.

- To use in a flu, cold, and tension bath, blend a few drops of orange essential oil with one teaspoon of carrier oil and a dispersant. Add to a warm bath to ease cold and flu symptoms.

- Add five drops of orange essential oil to one ounce of night cream or lotion to clarify skin.

- Orange essential oil supports collagen formation in mature skin. Add a few drops to one teaspoon of carrier oil and massage onto face and neck or area of concern.

- To liven your mood or relieve chronic anxiety, diffuse three drops of orange essential oil for thirty minutes, three times a day.

- To lift depression, put two drops of orange essential oil on a cotton ball and inhale four times a day.

---

5. Robert Tisserand and Rodney Young, *Essential Oils Safety second edition* (United Kingdom: Churchill Livingstone Elsevier, 2014), 371.

- For anxiety in children, diffuse three drops of orange essential oil in a diffuser no more than three minutes at a time. (Keep the diffuser twenty feet from the child.) Use three times a day to reduce symptoms.

- Diffuse orange essential oil to flush the body of toxins, gas, and bloating, and to help your body shed weight.

- For added energy, make an inhaler with two drops of lavender essential oil, one drop of peppermint essential oil, and three drops of orange essential oil. Use the inhaler five times a day.

- Orange essential oil can be used as a slug deterrent in your garden. Mix a few drops of orange essential oil in a spray bottle with one cup of water and spray plants to repel slugs. Shake well before use.

- Orange essential oil can be very helpful for IBS (irritable bowel syndrome) and other digestive issues. Mix two to three drops in one ounce of carrier oil such as olive or jojoba oil and massage on lower back and abdomen in a clockwise direction.

- For acne breakouts, moisten a cotton ball and add two drops of diluted orange essential oil. Dab lightly on acne and blemishes to remove excess facial oils.

- For joint and muscle pain, use two to three drops mixed in one teaspoon of carrier oil (jojoba, borage, flaxseed, olive) and massage on the affected area. (It can also be used with a hot compress.)

- To reduce skin inflammation associated with eczema and psoriasis, use two to three drops of orange essential oil in a carrier oil such as black seed, carrot seed, rose hip, grape seed, or jojoba and massage on the affected area.

- Relieve gingivitis and mouth ulcers by placing two to three drops of orange essential oil in a glass, then add water and mix. Swish in your mouth to cover the area but *do not* swallow. Repeat as often as needed.

Orange *(Citrus sinensis)* Essential Oil Blends Nicely With

Clove, eucalyptus, lavender, frankincense, sandalwood, and ylang-ylang essential oils.

fourteen

Patchouli *(Pogostemon cablin)* Essential Oil

Patchouli essential oil is a common ingredient in perfume and incense. The plant produces a conditioning oil with a heavy, pleasing, earthy scent. It was made famous in the 60s as a favorite oil of the hippie generation because it masked many odors associated with street living.

Patchouli *(Pogostemon cablin)* was named because of a native mint plant found in Madras which defined it as: *pach-chai* (green) + *ilai* (leaf). Patchouli grows well in warm and tropical climates. A bit fussy, it thrives in hot weather but not in direct sunlight. The seed-producing flowers are very fragrant and blossom in late fall.

Patchouli essential oil is affordable because it is frequently harvested and easily processed. Patchouli grows naturally in Southeast Asia. Its bushy plant is harvested several times a year by hand picking and the leaves are allowed to partially dry in the shade and ferment for a few days before the oil is steam extracted.

Patchouli is also one of the few essential oils that improves with age along with frankincense and sandalwood essential oils. A properly aged patchouli oil, like fine whiskey, is more desirable than a freshly bottled one.

Patchouli essential oil is classified as a sensual oil and may help people integrate their feelings when they seem out of touch with their bodies because it can relieve inhibition and assist with impotence and the fear of sex.

Patchouli essential oil may be an acquired taste for some. It was for me. It took me a long time to get used to the scent. I associated it with some negative memories as well as the scent of cheap imported clothing. As I learned to appreciate the scent, I started to appreciate the layers of the aroma. It's not something I want to diffuse for long, but every now and then I enjoy the warmth it brings to my heart and soul. I feel grounded when I diffuse it.

Mostly I use patchouli for its physical and medicinal qualities. The anti-inflammatory quality does wonders for a bruise, a bump, a sprain, or muscle aches. It is calming, settling, and does wonders for the skin. I have come to really cherish the healing properties of patchouli essential oil.

Source

Patchouli essential oil is obtained from the leaves and flowers of the *Pogostemon cablin* plant. Sometimes it can also be extracted using solvents. It has a strong, slightly sweet smell and you can detect musky, earthy, and dark overtones.

Benefits

Patchouli essential oil is digestive, anti-inflammatory, antifungal, antimicrobial, insecticidal, and relaxant. It has been popular in Asia and India for centuries. It has beneficial effects on skin and scalp conditions and is helpful in healing wounds and reducing the signs of scarring.

It is considered an excellent remedy for insect and snake bites and has been used as a fumigant. Because of its distinctive odor, patchouli essential oil is an antidepressant and mood lifter used to balance the body and stimulate a weakened immune system. It is said to bring into harmony the three principal forces at work within the body: the mind, body, and soul.

Precautions

Check in with your doctor before using patchouli essential oil if you are taking any blood-thinning or blood-clotting medications. Patchouli essential oil may inhibit blood clotting and could have interactions with drugs.

Creative Ways to Use Patchouli
(Pogostemon cablin) Essential Oil

- For an uplifting blend, use three drops of patchouli essential oil and one drop of rosemary essential oil. You can also place a few drops of this blend in an essential oil diffuser pendant necklace.

- Brighten your spirits by combining two drops of lemon essential oil, two drops of patchouli essential oil, and one drop of bergamot essential oil. This will uplift your mood and bring you the sense of joy. You can also diffuse or wear this blend.

- For sensual encouragement, mix one drop of geranium essential oil, one drop of patchouli essential oil, and one drop of bergamot essential oil. Diffuse or blend with a carrier oil and use as a massage oil blend.

- Add a few drops of patchouli essential oil to your favorite face cream or lotion to give skin a natural lift and improve your complexion.

- For help with eczema, mix a few drops of patchouli essential oil into one teaspoon of carrier oil like apricot seed or virgin olive oil and rub on affected areas.

- As a natural emotional balancer, mix three to four drops of patchouli essential oil with a carrier oil and use as a massage blend to help IBS when rubbed in a clockwise direction around the stomach and lower intestine.

Patchouli Essential Oil *(Pogostemon cablin)* Blends Nicely With

Rosemary, sandalwood, frankincense, bergamot, rose, citrus, clary sage, and rose geranium essential oils.

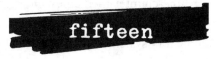

Peppermint *(Mentha x piperita)* Essential Oil

Peppermint is a cross between two types of mint: watermint and spearmint. It grows abundantly, similar to a weed, throughout Europe and North America. Ancient Egyptians used peppermint essential oil, based on the remnants of it found in the pyramids. In antiquity it also served many purposes for the Chinese and the Greeks, physically and emotionally.

Fancy chefs and home cooks have enjoyed the flavor and fragrance of the peppermint herb in main courses, salads, and desserts for centuries. Candies are flavored with peppermint, as are products like chewing gum, mints, ice creams, cough drops, tobacco, toothpaste, mouthwash, alcoholic beverages, detergents, soaps, and lipsticks. It is an active ingredient in over-the-counter medicines and digestive aids. Therapeutically, peppermint is used to treat many ailments of the skin, circulatory system, respiratory system, digestive system, immune system, and nervous system.

Cooling menthol is peppermint's most active ingredient, which is found in the leaves and flowers of the peppermint plant. The amount of menthol in a given plant is determined by the climate, habitat, and moisture in the soils.

I use peppermint essential oil to boost my energy level when I'm taking a long road trip, before and during workshops I teach, and lectures I give. You'll never see me reach for caffeine when I have peppermint essential oil handy. It works for nausea on a bumpy flight or a rocky boat trip. I use it in an inhaler when I travel abroad for keeping my stomach on track. I also combine it with lemon essential oil for a pick-me-up when I need more energy when I see clients or before a presentation. As the saying goes, I never leave home without it.

Source

Peppermint essential oil is steam distilled from the leaves, flowers, and buds.

Peppermint smells minty, fresh, cooling, herbal, and camphoric.

Benefits

Peppermint essential oil is used as a popular remedy for nausea, indigestion, cold symptoms, headaches, muscle and nerve pain, stomach aches, and intestinal conditions such as irritable bowel syndrome and stomach cramping. It is analgesic, a stimulant, combats flatulence, and works as a stomach tonic, an energy booster, mind clarifier, and performance enhancer.

Peppermint essential oil can also freshen breath, relieve headaches, improve mental focus, clear sinuses and the respiratory tract, lessen toothaches, provide headache relief, and even reduce fever.

Precautions

Peppermint essential oil contains menthol and as such may result in dizziness and nausea if inhaled at too strong a dose. People with gallbladder disease, severe liver damage, gallstones, and chronic heartburn should avoid the inhalation of peppermint essential oil.

Do not use in the first four months of pregnancy. Check the pregnancy guidelines for when it is safe for you to use peppermint essential oil.

Do not use on children under three years of age. Bronchial and respiratory stress can occur in infants and adults by using too strong a mixture on chest and nasal areas. Never apply undiluted peppermint essential oil to feet or put on children under age the age of twelve.

Creative Ways to Use Peppermint
(Mentha x piperita) Essential Oil

- To relieve stomach ache, massage several drops of peppermint essential oil, diluted with a carrier oil, on your abdomen in a clockwise motion.

- Place a drop of diluted peppermint essential oil on wrists, or inhale to soothe motion sickness or general nausea. Dilute according to your skin sensitivity.

- Use peppermint essential oil, diluted in a carrier oil, to massage and soothe an aching back, sore muscles, and melt away tension headaches.

- One study[6] found that peppermint essential oil, mixed with eucalyptus essential oil and capsaicin, the active ingredient in chili peppers, may be helpful for the relief of pain. Topically apply diluted peppermint essential oil to relieve pain associated with fibromyalgia and myofascial pain syndrome.

- Inhaling diffused peppermint essential oil can unclog your sinuses and offer relief from a scratchy throat.

- Diffused or inhaled as a steam, a few drops of peppermint essential oil can act as an expectorant and may provide the relief you need for colds, cough, sinusitis, asthma, and bronchitis.

- Apply a few drops of peppermint essential oil mixed with lavender essential oil and diluted in a carrier oil to achy joints to cool muscles like an ice while the rest of you stays warm.

- Inhale peppermint essential oil to stave off the munchies. If you don't have a diffuser with you at dinnertime, apply a couple of diluted drops to your temples or chest, or take a couple of deep sniffs from a few

---

6. Chakrabordy, HC Chandola and Arunangschu, *Fibromyalgia and Myofascial Pain Syndrome-A Dilemma.* Oct 5, 2009. Accessed Dec 23, 2018. https://www.ncbi.nlm.nih.gov/pmc/articles/PMC2900090/#CIT21.

drops diluted in your palms and rubbed together to release the essential oil molecules. (You can easily make a portable inhaler to use as an appetite suppressant.) The minty aroma helps curb your appetite.

- For an energy boost, take a few whiffs of peppermint essential oil. It will perk you up on long road trips, in school, at classes, or at those times when you're tired and need a jolt of natural energy.

- Dilute and rub in your palms before sniffing for a quicker picker-upper.

- When diffused, two to three drops of peppermint essential oil may improve focus and concentration.

- Add two to three drops of peppermint essential oil to your regular shampoo and conditioner to stimulate the scalp and help remove dandruff. Do not fill the whole bottle. Use one dose at a time.

- Inhaled or diffused, peppermint essential oil can relax the muscles in your nasal passages and help clear out the congestion and pollen during allergy season.

- Diffusing peppermint essential oil mixed with clove bud essential oil and eucalyptus essential oil can also reduce seasonal allergy symptoms. The same mix works well in an inhaler to fend off reactions during allergy season.

- Inhale diluted peppermint essential oil to help curb your appetite by triggering a sense of fullness thus curbing your cravings.

Peppermint *(Mentha x piperita)*
Essential Oil Blends Nicely With

Basil, eucalyptus, rose geranium, lavender, lemon, rosemary and tea tree essential oils.

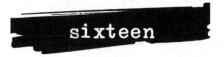

Pine *(Pinus sylvestris)* Essential Oil

P ine is a common scent used in cleaning products around the world. Known also as an all-around healer, pine *(Pinus sylvestris)* essential oil comes from trees known as Scotch pine, Norway pine, and Forest pine. The trees are strong and tall and so is the essential oil, which is derived via steam distillation from the needles, twigs, and stumps of the tree.

Pine essential oil is rich in monoterpenes, which makes it a superior cleanser, purifier, disinfectant, and deodorizer. The oil is used in soaps, disinfectants, and in rosin for violin strings. The next time you attend a symphony orchestra event, you'll know pine had a lot to do with the melodious sound of the string section.

As far back as ancient Egypt, cooks used the kernels of the pine tree for cooking. (Pine nuts, anyone?) The Scotch pine can live for 750 years. Native Americans stuffed their mattresses with pine needles to ward off fleas, lice, and other creepy crawlers. It is also used by gardeners to repel slugs and snails.

Positioning a bough of pine branches over the entrance to a house invited joy within the walls in Japanese culture. In other cultures, pine cones were burned inside the hearth during the winter to purify and cleanse the air. Northern cultures used pine to cultivate a vigorous old age.

The Romans used it for muscle aches and respiratory problems. Nordic peoples used it to purify the air in their homes during the winter months. Pine essential oil has been used as a winter wellness staple for hundreds of years across many civilizations and generations.

Because pine essential oil is 90 percent monoterpenes, it oxidizes quickly and should be stored in the refrigerator when not being used.

I chose to include pine in this book because it has a common, familiar, foresty scent. I like to use it around the house because I've never run across anyone who doesn't enjoy the fresh smell of pine.

I grew up in the Pacific Northwest, so I was very familiar with pine. Pine brings back wonderful memories. Winters were filled with the burning of pine logs and the cutting of Christmas trees. The very scent of pine takes me back to those snow-covered streets when life was simpler, and the smell of chocolate chip cookies wafted out of Nana's kitchen on the way home from school. I almost feel like I am ten again whenever I diffuse pine essential oil. Almost.

Source

Pine essential oil is steam distilled from stumps, twigs, needles, and cones of pine trees. It has a clean, healthy, and invigorating scent.

Benefits

Pine essential oil is antifungal, antimicrobial, antibacterial, anti-inflammatory, has antiseptic properties, and is a disinfectant. This essential oil is good for the entire body.

It can be very helpful with rheumatism and arthritis because it can be applied to areas of inflammation to soothe and calm the pain by reducing swelling. It can be an emotionally uplifting scent when diffused.

Precautions

Do not use if you are prone to skin allergies or allergic reactions of the skin. Be sure to perform a patch test before using. Do not use on infants and do not take internally.

Creative Ways to Use Pine
(Pinus sylvestris) Essential Oil

- For facial fatigue, use four drops of pine essential oil in one ounce of lotion and massage into the muscles of your face.

- To help relieve a stuffy nose and chest cold, add two drops each of pine, eucalyptus, lemon, rosemary, marjoram, and thyme essential oils properly dispersed in a pot of steaming water. Turn off the heat, place a towel over your head to cover the pot, close your eyes, and inhale for three to five minutes.

- To make a purifying house cleaning spray, add twelve drops each of pine, eucalyptus, tea tree, and thyme essential oil to a twelve-ounce bottle of water. Shake well and spray the room. Make sure pets and children are not present because these are strong essential oils. You can use the same mixture to clean counter tops and surfaces and to disinfect sick rooms.

- For a boost of strength and vitality, diffuse three to four drops of pine essential oil.

- Apply a compress of pine essential oil to achy joints or inflamed muscles. Use two to four drops on a cloth diluted in a carrier oil such as emu, olive, borage, flaxseed, or jojoba for best results.

- Use as a rub for arthritic and inflamed joints. Mix with a carrier oil (emu, olive, borage, flaxseed, or jojoba) and apply to the area of pain.

- To soothe a burn, mix two drops of pine essential oil in one teaspoon of castor oil and apply to the burn.

- For relieving a headache, drop two drops of pine essential oil onto a cotton ball and sniff five times. Wait thirty seconds and sniff again. Repeat this process for two minutes. Your headache should be lessened.

- Use a few drops of pine essential oil in garbage pails for freshness and purifying.

Pine *(Pinus sylvestris)* Essential Oil Blends Nicely With

Citrus oils like lemon, bergamot, orange, lavender, eucalyptus, frankincense, sandalwood, tea tree, and thyme essential oils.

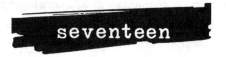
Rose *(Rosa x damascena)* Essential Oil

T he rose flower is associated with love, feelings of romance, beauty, and the color red. The rose has captivated humankind for sixty million years, according to the discovery of ancient fossilized roses. The first rose came from Asia during the Eocene epoch and they now hail from gardens around the world. The Damask rose, *Rosa x damascena*, comes from gardens in Bulgaria, Turkey, the Middle East, China, and Russia. The Cabbage rose, *Rosa centifolia*, is farmed in France, Morocco, and Egypt. Most rose essential oil is made from the Damask rose. Originally, the rose oil was used in perfumes, but it has evolved into far more uses.

Rose essential oil has been used throughout history in the ancient art of aromatherapy as a healing tonic and mood-elevating supplement. The Benedictine Monks grew and preserved roses in their apothecary gardens using them for medicinal purposes during the Middle Ages in Europe, even when herbal healing was banned by the Catholic Church.

In the tenth century, a Persian physician and philosopher, Avicenna, chose the rose as the first plant for his new distillery. His distillery continued to be in constant use for six centuries in Shiraz and they manufactured millions of bottles of rose essential oil during those millennia.

Rose petals are not very high in oil content: a rose blossom contains only about 0.02 percent essential oil, therefore it requires 60,000 roses to produce just one ounce of oil, or ten thousand pounds of rose blossoms to produce one pound of oil. As a result of the immense quantity of blossoms required for production, rose essential oil tends to be expensive. However, its price does not prevent it from being one of the most popular essential oils available.

Rose essential oil comes in two main types: rose absolute and rose otto. They are both used for the same purposes. Rose essential oil otto is said to be the best type of rose essential oil for aromatherapy because it is extremely heady. One can use much less in a blend with other essential oils and it seems to keep longer than rose absolute. The color of rose absolute tends to be a dark orange to red with an intense, pungent rosey aroma. It is preferred by perfumers and is said to be closer in fragrance to the flower than an otto. Only your experience with each of them will determine your preference of the rose otto or rose absolute.

Rose is very important in my life. I truly cherish this essential oil, and if I have one splurge it's on rose absolute or otto essential oil. Rose essential oil has soothed many heartaches for me and put me to sleep during stressful times.

In 2017, I was evacuated during the Thomas Fire in Ventura, California. The approaching flames were eighty feet tall and I had barely seven minutes to get out of the house with seven pets. In that seven minutes, all I could grab were my pets and their carriers. I was in my nightgown and slippers, with nothing else but my purse and cellphone, which I grabbed on my way out the door for what I thought might be the last time. I drove away in fear for my life.

The next day, after buying some clothes and underwear, my next stop was the health food store where I purchased some basic supplies and a few essential oils. One of them was rose. I knew my heart needed mending after such a fright. I waited for three days before I knew if we had a house or not. On television I watched the homes of my neighbors burn to the ground in front of my eyes. Those were desperate and frightening hours. Rose essential oil helped me deal with the emotions of not knowing the outcome of my fate.

Source

Rose essential oil is extracted from the petals of various types of roses. *Rose ottos* are extracted from the petals through steam distillation, while *rose absolutes* are obtained through solvent extraction of the blossoms. Rose has a sweet floral and rich scent. The color of a rose will determine its scent.

Benefits

Damask rose essential oil soothes and harmonizes the mind and helps lift depression. It quells anger, alleviates grief, and reduces fear, nervous tension, headaches, and stress. It promotes self-nurturing, self-esteem, and solving emotional problems. It has the properties of being an antidepressant, antiseptic, antiviral, aphrodisiac, astringent, and a laxative. It has been shown to be beneficial to the liver and stomach, and can repair broken capillaries, reduce inflammation and skin redness, and is useful for eczema and herpes. It can also help regulate the circulatory system.

Rose essential oil's greatest benefit is that it unites the physical with the emotional by healing imbalances that may exist between the body, mind, and spirit.

Precautions

Rose essential oil is non-toxic, non-irritant, and non-sensitizing, but should not be used during pregnancy without the proper supervision of a credentialed Aromatherapist.

Creative Ways to Rose
(Rosa x damascena) Essential Oil

- For acne, dab one drop of pure diluted rose essential oil on blemishes three times a day. Make sure you use a sterile cotton swab. If the antimicrobial power is too much for you, dilute it again with a carrier oil. Never apply neat.
- Diffuse rose essential oil to help poor circulation and heart problems such as arrhythmia and high blood

pressure. It can also be diffused or inhaled to boost liver and gall bladder functions.

- Diffuse a few drops of rose essential oil for relief from asthma, coughs, hay fever, digestive system disorders, and for liver congestion and nausea.

- Diffuse rose essential oil for clearing, cleansing, and regulating female sex organs and hormones. It provides an overall toning effect on the uterus.

- Rose essential oil is excellent for dry, mature, and irritated skin. Add a few drops to your favorite cream or moisturizer along with a drop or two of sandalwood essential oil.

- Diffused or inhaled, rose essential oil provides a feeling of well-being and happiness; it also calms a nervous or anxious mind.

- Diffused, rose essential oil can ease allergies, asthma, baby blues, headaches, migraine, and nervous tension.

- Diffused or inhaled, a few drops of rose essential oil can help reduce feelings of depression, anger, and grief while dealing with emotional problems such as sadness and loss. It is a great tonic for matters of the heart.

- To reduce skin redness, fight inflammations, and fix broken capillaries, use a few drops of rose essential oil mixed with one teaspoon of a carrier oil and massage into skin. Nice results have been achieved for light varicose veins.

Rose *(Rosa x damascena)*
Essential Oil Blends Nicely With

Bergamot, Roman chamomile, clary sage, rose geranium, lavender, lemon, patchouli, sandalwood, and ylang-ylang essential oils.

eighteen

Roman Chamomile (*Chamaemelum nobile*) Essential Oil

R oman chamomile was one of the nine sacred oils of the Saxons. The word chamomile is derived from Greek— *chamos* (ground) and *melos* (apple), referring to the fact that the plant grows low to the ground, and the fresh blooms have a pleasing apple scent and flavor. The Spaniards called it *Manzanilla*, (little apple), and gave the same name to one of their sherries, which they flavored with this aromatic plant.[7]

The early Egyptians, Greeks, and Romans reportedly used it widely for its gentle, healing qualities. The English

---

7. "Chamomille," herbs-info.com, http://www.herbs-info.com/chamomile. html accessed 10/2/2015 n.d.

used it in the pot for stews, and the Spanish used it to flavor their vintages of sherry. Some use it for dyeing fabrics.

If you step on the growing plant, chamomile releases a strong and potent airborne smell. Legend has it that nothing contributes so much to the health of a garden as a number of chamomile plants dispersed around. If one of the other plants is drooping and sickly, it is said to recover if you place a chamomile plant or even a cutting near it. I was fascinated by this claim that the chamomile plant can aid another sickly plant and bring it back to life when planted next to it in the garden. By Jove it does! I tried it several times and the chamomile plant is a real lifesaver. Chamomile is a born healer in the garden and beyond.

There are two different types of chamomile essential oil: *Roman chamomile* and *German blue chamomile*. I feature the Roman chamomile here. But the German blue is also wonderful and has excellent qualities. I'll discuss both because as a beginner it can be easy to confuse them when you purchase your oil. Learning about the characteristics of both will help you understand the benefits of each. German blue chamomile essential oil is about double the cost of Roman chamomile.

Roman chamomile calms the nervous system and suppresses anxiety and stress. It contains esters, which are chemicals that have antispasmodic qualities that can alleviate digestive cramping and discomfort.

German blue chamomile is excellent for easing pain and for assisting the nasal passage with allergies. It also helps with minor cuts and abrasions and soothes frayed nerves, delivering a good night's sleep.

I like the calming, soothing, and healing benefits of everyday Roman chamomile essential oil. It's a pleasant way to end the day or take a relaxing break from the stress of work. Diffusing a few drops relaxes me after a long day. Too much though, and I want to make an early night of it! I prefer to use diffused Roman chamomile to unwind even before I start to make dinner. I feel more grounded and more apt to choose healthier fare when I'm not still wound up from work.

Source

Roman chamomile oil is obtained through steam distillation of the *Chamaemelum nobile* plant flowers.

Benefits

Anti-inflammatory, analgesic, nervine (stress reliever), relaxant, and sedative, this essential oil is all-around amazing. Roman chamomile *(Chamaemelum nobile)* essential oil helps to decrease gas (flatulence), relax muscles, and treat hay fever, inflammation, rheumatism, muscle spasms, PMS, menstrual disorders, insomnia, ulcers, gastrointestinal disorders, hemorrhoids, nervousness, joint stiffness, and muscular aches and pains. It also relieves dry, itchy skin, puffiness, and some allergenic skin conditions. Known as a skin aid, it can heal blisters and improve elasticity and tissue strength. It has even been used to lighten fair hair.

Precautions

Avoid using Roman chamomile essential oil if you are pregnant or breastfeeding.

Roman chamomile essential oil can cause an allergic reaction in people who are sensitive to ragweed, chrysanthemums, marigolds, daisies, and others. Do not use without checking with your physician if you have allergies to these plants.

Creative Ways to Use Roman Chamomile (*Chamaemelum nobile*) Essential Oil

- Roman chamomile essential oil can be applied topically, as a compress, in the bath (properly dispersed), through direct inhalation, or a few drops in a diffuser.

- Add a few drops of properly dispersed Roman chamomile essential oil to bathwater before bedtime to bring about a calm, peaceful sleep.

- Diffuse Roman chamomile essential oil or apply several diluted drops to the soles of your feet to reduce fever and calm frayed nerves.

- For an anti-inflammatory, mix together three drops of Roman chamomile essential oil, three drops of helichrysum essential oil, two drops of sandalwood essential oil, and two drops of lavender essential oil in one ounce of carrier oil and apply topically as needed.

- To make a gentle bath for all ages, add two drops of Roman chamomile essential oil and two drops of lavender essential oil to warm bathwater. Disperse properly and dilute with coconut, rice, or almond milk.

- Diluted with a carrier oil, it can be massaged in or mixed with a few drops of carrier oil and placed in a warm cloth to use as a compress for headaches.

- Diffuse a few drops of fragrant Roman chamomile essential oil to ease headaches and nervous tension.

- Add one to two drops of Roman chamomile essential oil to your favorite moisturizer, shampoo, or conditioner to promote youthful looking skin and hair.

- Add drops of Roman chamomile essential oil in a steam bath and inhale it for sinus inflammation, hay fever, sore throat, ear inflammation, and as a painkiller.

- For supple skin, add Roman chamomile essential oil to your face or body lotion, or use a very small amount of essential oil mixed with a carrier oil like carrot seed, rose hip, jojoba, pomegranate, sweet almond, or tamanu.

- For a calming and restorative salve, combine one half cup pure virgin coconut oil with one quarter cup beeswax and heat on low or medium heat until mixed. Be careful not to burn the mixture. During the cooling process, stir in fifteen drops each of Roman chamomile essential oil and lavender essential oil.

- Adding a few drops of Roman chamomile essential oil mixed with one teaspoon of carrier oil to bathwater and correctly dispersed (chapter 4) can ease inflammation of the skin and soothe a sunburn.

- For restful sleep, combine witch hazel, ten drops each of Roman chamomile essential oil and lavender essential oil, and five drops of orange essential oil in a four-ounce spray bottle. Shake well. Spray on linens before bed for more restful sleep. (Pretest linens to make sure they don't stain.)

Roman Chamomile *(Chamaemelum nobile)* Essential Oil Blends Nicely With

Bergamot, clary sage, eucalyptus, rose geranium, grapefruit, lavender, lemon, rose, tea tree, and ylang-ylang essential oils.

nineteen

Rose Geranium *(Pelargonium graveolens)* Essential Oil

The name for the plant rose geranium, *Pelargonium graveolens,* comes from the Greek *pelargos,* which means *stork.* The word *graveolens* refers to the strong-smelling leaves. This definition is specific to *Geranium pelargonium,* also known as rose-scented geranium, which is one of the few known species of flower that is safe for human consumption. The flowers vary from pale pink to almost white, and the leaves may be strongly rose-scented.

Rose geranium may hail from southern Africa, but it has become a cheery garden plant throughout the world. They were brought to Europe in the seventeenth century. Versatile geranium essential oil not only boasts health benefits, but it is also used in making perfumes, soaps, detergents, and household products. Geranium essential oil has been described more than once as a natural perfume.

The rose geranium plant is vulnerable to the climate and soil in which it grows. Much like a quartz crystal that turns yellow when it grows near sulphur, the geranium takes on the characteristics of its neighbors and the organic medium it is planted in. Because of that amazing chameleon-like talent, geranium essential oil can range from very sweet and rosy to musty, minty, and greenish.

Geraniums originally earned their popularity in gardens and as balcony plants because of their insect-repellant properties. Geranium essential oil can now be found as a main ingredient in commercial insect repellant preparations, joining ranks with fellow essential oils like bergamot, lemon, and citronella. Room sprays prepared with geranium essential oil help to keep your house insect free in summer.

You will see rose geranium essential oil sold as geranium essential oil and listed with bourbon in the name. They are the same thing. Bourbon delineates that the essential oil comes from the Réunion Islands. It does not mean drink this at parties. That kind of bourbon comes from Kentucky.

In contrast to ylang-ylang essential oil, which may be considered heavy, rose geranium is light, sweet, and floral without being overly heady. Depending on where the geranium plant comes from and the mineral content of the soil, it will have different smells not only by region, but year after year due to the change in the soil's chemical content or how much rain the region had. It's like a chameleon in the way that it changes to fit its environment. I like to consider this a strength because it makes the geranium essential oil full of new surprises each time I purchase a bottle.

If you are into angels and angel healing, this essential oil is definitely angelic. Its aroma and viscosity is heavenly in nature and practice. I like using this oil for counseling sessions when there is tension in the air or disagreement. Without saying a thing, this scent permeates the air, detoxifies it physically and emotionally, and quells rising anger and hostility. It's not an offensive aroma at all, but a very neutral one, so it's hardly noticed. Because of its subtlety, it is a powerful agent for transformation.

Source

Rose geranium essential oil is steam distilled from the flowers, leaves, and stalks of the plant (also known as the aerial parts). It has a light, sweet, and floral scent and is often substituted for the more costly rose essential oil.

Benefits

Rose geranium essential oil is anti-inflammatory, anticancerous, antibacterial, antifungal, astringent, and vulnerary (wound healing).

It can help improve skin conditions such as dermatitis, eczema, and psoriasis. It has been known to improve blood flow; stimulate the liver and pancreas; help detox the liver; cleanse oily skin; and attack tough infections like ringworm, herpes, and shingles. Rose geranium essential oil has been used to relieve stress and depression, reduce inflammation and irritation, and improve the overall health of the skin. Many women claim it alleviates the effects of menopause.

Precautions

Geranium essential oil influences certain hormone secretions and is therefore not advised for use by pregnant women or those who are breastfeeding. Tisserand and Young[8] advise a maximum dermal concentration of 17.5 percent.

Creative Ways to Use Rose Geranium (*Pelargonium graveolens*) Essential Oil

- For PMS relief, blend one teaspoon geranium essential oil in two ounces of carrier oil and apply to breasts to ease soreness and swelling.

- For softer and more supple skin, add a few drops of geranium essential oil to bathwater diluted in a dispersant, mix with a carrier oil to apply to skin, or add a few drops to your facial cream.

- Diffuse three drops of geranium essential oil to disinfect room air and create a pleasant environment.

- For tension and stress relief, add three drops of geranium essential oil to one teaspoon of carrier oil for a massage solution to help circulation and tonify the liver. It also helps relieve tightness.

- For cold sores, place one drop of diluted geranium essential oil on a cotton swab and dab the affected area.

- As a mood balancer, diffuse two to three drops, or place two drops of geranium essential oil on a cotton ball or handkerchief and inhale deeply two to three times. Pause and repeat.

---

8. Robert Tisserand and Rodney Young, *Essential Oils Safety second edition* (United Kingdom: Churchill Livingstone Elsevier, 2014), 293.

- For headache and pain relief, add eight to ten drops of geranium essential oil mixed with one tablespoon dispersant in bathwater to help relieve headache, PMS, stress, and tension.

- To dispel cellulite, mix twenty drops of geranium essential oil in one ounce of carrier oil and massage on the body, focusing on the lower back.

- To repel mosquitos, diffuse five to six drops of geranium essential oil mixed with two drops of eucalyptus essential oil for a strong repellent.

- Relieve insomnia caused by stress by placing four drops of geranium essential oil on a tissue or cotton ball and place inside your pillowcase. Or you can diffuse two to three drops of geranium essential oil.

- For respiratory problems, use five drops of geranium essential oil in a vaporizer or diffuser.

- For a sore throat and tonsillitis relief, use two to five drops of geranium essential oil in a steam inhalation. Or put two drops of geranium essential oil in a glass of warm water and gargle. Do not swallow.

- For use as an aphrodisiac, use eight to ten drops of geranium essential oil in a bath (use proper dispersant) or use two to three drops in a diffuser. For more variety, you can add in a few drops of patchouli essential oil or sandalwood essential oil to the diffuser to enrich the blend.

Rose Geranium *(Pelargonium graveolens)* Essential Oil Blends Nicely With

Bergamot, lavender, orange, lemon, ylang-ylang, clary sage, rose, sandalwood, and rosemary essential oils.

twenty

Rosemary
(Rosmarinus officinalis)
Essential Oil

The name rosemary derives from Latin for "dew" (*ros*) and "sea" (*marinus*), or dew of the sea. The Romans used rosemary in religious ceremonies and for blessings at weddings. Rosemary was an all-around herb for the ancients. They gave it special importance and used it in food preparation, cosmetic care, and for medicinal purposes. The Romans weren't the first to capture its fragrance, though. The ancient Egyptians cornered its qualities long before and used it as an aromatic incense for their worship rituals.

The herb rosemary is very popular in countries and cultures around the Mediterranean. The rosemary bush is part of the mint family, which includes basil, lavender, myrtle, and sage.

Regional dishes are cooked with rosemary oil and garnished with freshly plucked rosemary leaves. The stems and branches of the plant can be used to cook foods in an outdoor barbeque, allowing the flavor and smoke from the wood to permeate the food. Soak the branches in water and wrap in aluminum foil. Poke air holes in the foil and place the foil packets of stems and branches on the coals. The steam and smoke from the branches will flavor the food you grill.

Paracelsus, renowned German-Swiss physician and botanist, made significant contributions to the understanding of herbal medicine during the sixteenth century. He valued rosemary essential oil because of its ability to strengthen the entire body. He used it extensively because he discovered that rosemary essential oil had the ability to heal delicate organs such as the liver, brain, and heart.

When selecting your rosemary essential oil, there is one area to be mindful of: chemotypes, which means a variation of the plant type. Rosemary has six variations. We will address the three major ones. Each chemotype brings with it different healing properties and potential sensitivities. The chemotype is abbreviated as "ct." Note: ct. verbenone or ct. 1,8-cineole are the safest to use.

Rosmarinus officinalis ct. camphor is high in ketones and works best for muscle aches and pains, massage relief, addresses rheumatism discomfort, and has diuretic and circulatory benefits. Camphor can be neurotoxic if the essential oil contains high levels of it.

Rosmarinus officinalis ct. 1,8-cineole is high in oxides. It is antiviral, antifungal, antibacterial, and anti-inflammatory. It is the better choice for alleviating respiratory and mucous issues. Added to shampoo, it can restore vitality to dull hair and works as a blood stimulator when massaged into the head.

Rosmarinus officinalis ct. verbenone is best used on the skin because it contains ketones and monoterpenes, which inhibit the accumulation of toxins. It bears antispasmodic benefits and is antibacterial, anti-depressive, antirheumatic, and expectorant. It can also be used successfully for respiratory issues.

If all that sounds too confusing, just remember to focus on what you want to solve and then back into your choice by checking out which chemotype suits your specific needs.

Ever since I lived in France for a year, my hobby has been cooking international foods. You can't help but be influenced by the seasonal vegetables and herbs available in the neighborhood markets. I experimented with everything I could find. Rosemary has become a main staple.

Source

Rosemary essential oil is most commonly extracted through steam distillation of the plant's flowering tops and leaves. In some instances, the leaves can be cold pressed. Rosemary brings a clean, crisp, fresh herbaceous smell to the party.

Benefits

Rosemary essential oil is an astringent, analgesic, diuretic, memory enhancer, antirheumatic, tonic, stimulant, and excellent detoxifier.

It is known to be restorative, purifying, protective, reviving, and refreshing. Rosemary essential oil contributes relief to aching muscles, arthritis, dull skin, exhaustion, gout, dandruff, hair and scalp thinning, neuralgia, poor circulation, acne, impaired memory, and helps with weight loss.

Precautions

Rosemary essential oil should not be used by pregnant women. Essential oil authorities Tisserand and Young warn us that rosemary oil can be neurotoxic if it contains a high level of camphor.[9] Do not use on or near the face of infants and children.

Creative Ways to Use Rosemary (*Rosmarinus officinalis*) Essential Oil

- If you are looking to improve your memory, mix three drops of rosemary (ct. 1,8-cineole) essential oil with one teaspoon of pure essential oil and rub on your upper neck or diffuse alone for one hour a day.

- If your hair is thinning, or you'd like to control your dandruff, use rosemary (ct. 1,8-cineole) essential oil as a hair thickener. Massage five drops of diluted rosemary (ct. 1,8-cineole) essential oil onto your scalp after each shower.

---

9. Robert Tisserand and Rodney Young, *Essential Oils Safety second edition* (United Kingdom: Churchill Livingstone Elsevier, 2014), 409.

- To reduce joint and muscle pain, mix two drops of rosemary (ct. camphor or ct. verbenone) essential oil, two drops of peppermint essential oil, and one tablespoon of carrier oil (borage, flaxseed, or Emu) and rub onto sore muscles and painful joints.

- Used externally, rosemary (ct. camphor or ct. verbenone) essential oil can help soothe the stomach and relieve pain from indigestion, menstrual cramps, or other difficulties. Dilute in a carrier oil and rub onto torso in a clockwise motion.

- To assist gallbladder function, mix three drops of rosemary (ct. 1,8-cineole) essential oil with one teaspoon of carrier oil and massage clockwise over gallbladder area twice daily.

- To relieve neuropathy and neuralgia discomfort, add two drops of rosemary (ct. 1,8-cineole) essential oil to three drops of helichrysum essential oil, three drops of cypress essential oil, and one tablespoon of a carrier oil and rub on area of neuropathy.

- Rub rosemary essential oil (ct. verbenone) on your feet, temples, or wrists (or anywhere) to bring about an immediate calming effect throughout your whole body. Dilute in a carrier oil.

- Add a few drops of rosemary essential oil to a dryer sheet to deodorize and freshen your laundry. (A wet cloth works just as well.)

- Diffusing a few drops of rosemary essential oil (ct. verbenone or ct. 1,8-cineole) aids circulation, liver function, and, as a stimulant, encourages weight loss.

- For super-effective weight loss, make an inhaler and use it five times a day to discourage appetite. I suggest rosemary, black pepper, and pink grapefruit to help quell appetite. (Follow the inhaler instructions in chapter 26.)

Rosemary *(Rosmarinus officinalis)* Essential Oil Blends Nicely With

Frankincense, lavender, clary sage, thyme, Roman chamomile, and peppermint essential oils.

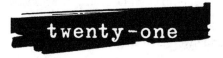

twenty-one

Sandalwood *(Santalum album)* Essential Oil

S andalwood, also known by its nickname *Liquid Gold*, is an evergreen tree that is native to southern Asia. The oil comes from the heartwood of the tree. Sandalwood was first recorded in AD 78 by Dioscorides in *De Materia Medica*, a book filled with descriptions of hundreds of plants and herbs. This book was used as the standard reference until sometime in the seventeenth century.

Sandalwood essential oil has a distinctive soft, warm, smooth, creamy, and milky precious-wood scent. It has been used for centuries and, among other sacred uses, it has been said that it was used by the ancient east Indians when they built their ancient edifices. They used sandalwood essential oils to perfume the mortar between the bricks. Hence, as you approached the temple, it knocked you over with the aroma and prepared you for something sacred.

True sandalwoods belong to the same botanical family as European mistletoe. Indian sandalwood (*Santalum album*) and Australian sandalwood (*Santalum spicatum*) head the list of desirable producers. It is ecologically important to distinguish between the different sandalwood essential oils on the market. The original source of true sandalwood, *Santalum album*, is Indian.

Sandalwood is a protected species, and current demand for it cannot be adequately met. The genus *Santalum* has more than nineteen species. Some avaricious traders try to pawn off these other species as the real deal, but they are not. Most of the substitute woods are substandard and quickly lose their aroma. It's best to stay with Indian sandalwood essential oil products as long as they are fairly traded and responsibly harvested by growers who renew their assets.

Santalum album trees in India are now owned by the government in order to monitor the illegal harvesting of the trees. The Indian government controls 75 percent of the total output of sandalwood in the world. The legal harvesting mandate is: a sandalwood tree should be at least fifteen years old before it is cut down. Illegal tree-poaching is a recurring national problem because sadly, many trees get the axe well before their time, often in the dead of night, thus creating a product in the marketplace that is inferior as well as harming the prospects for the future of sandalwoods.

Historians say that ancient Egyptians imported the wood and used it for medicines, embalming, and ritual burnings to venerate their gods. Sandalwood essential oil was believed to promote spiritual practices, peaceful relaxation, openness, and grounding. It is still used in many funeral ceremonies to help the dead cross over and as a comfort for the mourners. Traditionally, it's been used in many initiation rites to open the disciple's mind when he is about to receive consecration.

Sandalwood is another essential oil I find centering, grounding, and uplifting at the same time. I feel wise when I diffuse it and I will often wear it in a pendant to keep me emotionally even-keeled if I need to sit through a long meeting or a discussion that might have dissonance involved.

Sandalwood is in almost all the cosmetic creams I make and use. It's also a great repellant. I use a small diffuser out in the garden when I want to sit outside with a cup of tea and enjoy the backyard. It keeps me and my plants free of unwanted flying visitors.

Source

Sandalwood oil is achieved through steam distillation, hydro distillation, or CO_2 extraction of the wood of the tree. CO_2 produces a darker and less aromatic oil. Sandalwood essential oil smells lightly powdery, warm, and sometimes like creamy wood.

Benefits

Sandalwood essential oil is an astringent, disinfectant, stimulant, tonic, antidepressant, antibacterial, antiviral, and immune stimulant. It is a calming, grounding, stabilizing, sacred, aphrodisiac. Sandalwood essential oil is also helpful with skin repair. As a relaxant it is very effective for urogenital and pulmonary disorders, viral infections, cold sores, and herpes simplex.

Precautions

Breastfeeding mothers and young children should avoid using sandalwood essential oil. The oil can cause an allergic skin reaction in certain individuals, so it is important to first patch test on a small area of skin. Japanese people can have photoallergic reactions to doses over 2 percent dilution.[10]

Creative Ways to Use Sandalwood
(Santalum album) Essential Oil

- Diffuse a few drops of sandalwood essential oil at bed time to relax and de-stress before sleep.
- Apply several drops of diluted sandalwood essential oil on strained locations like ankles and wrists (be sure to patch test first).
- Directly inhale fumes of sandalwood essential oil from a two-drop-soaked cotton ball for relaxation.
- Three to four drops of sandalwood essential oil added to a vaporizer is romantically effective and an aphrodisiac.
- Use a few drops of sandalwood essential oil in an inhaler to clear bronchitis, coughs, chest infections, asthma, irritability, nervous tension, and stress.

---

10. Robert Tisserand and Rodney Young, *Essential Oils Safety second edition* (United Kingdom: Churchill Livingstone Elsevier, 2014), 418.

- Use a few drops of sandalwood essential oil in a vaporizer to ward off bugs and act as an automatic insect repellant.

- Use a few drops of sandalwood essential oil mixed with a proper dispersant in bathwater to alleviate bladder infections and scar tissue, and improve eczema and stretch marks.

- Add a few drops of sandalwood essential oil to your favorite lotion or cream to assist with chapped, dry, or inflamed skin. Sandalwood essential oil has wonderful moisturizing and hydrating properties that are great for antiaging skin care.

- For wrinkles, massage one to two drops of diluted sandalwood essential oil directly into the area of concern. Dilute lightly with a moisturizer or carrier oil like argan, borage, macadamia nut, neem, or tamanu.

- Use diluted sandalwood essential oil mixed with one ounce of pure water as a toner for aiding oily skin. Shake well each time you use.

- For an at-home facial, fill a large bowl with steaming water, then apply one to two drops of diluted sandalwood essential oil (make sure you do a patch test first) to your face and cover head with a towel. Place your face over the steaming water for five to ten minutes. Your skin will feel nourished and rejuvenated.

- To help restore moisture and give hair a silky shine, apply one to two drops of diluted sandalwood essential oil to wet hair.

• To lessen tension and balance your emotions, place two drops of diluted sandalwood essential oil directly into your palms and rub together, then inhale. Or you can diffuse for the same results.

Sandalwood *(Santalum album)* Essential Oil Blends Nicely With

Bergamot, rose geranium, lavender, rose, and ylang-ylang essential oils.

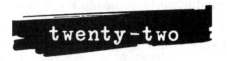
twenty-two

Tea Tree *(Melaleuca alternifolia)* Essential Oil

Tea tree was named by a group of eighteenth-century sailors who made a pot of tea from the leaves of a tree they found when they came ashore on the south coast of Australia. It smelled to them like nutmeg, so they called it tea tree.

This *Melaleuca alternifolia* tree is native to Australia, specifically Queensland and New South Wales, and its oil has been known and used among the indigenous people as a universal medicinal remedy since ancient times. Aborigines in the area ground up the leaves to make a salve for skin wounds. The leaves are also used as an herbal tea to help cure respiratory ailments. Early travelers to Australia spread the word about the healing properties of the plant in the 1920s and suddenly the world wanted to know more. For more than ninety years, numerous studies have tested tea tree essential oil's effects on skin ailments, infections, and rashes and have concluded that it is a potentially viable treatment for certain conditions.

The characterization of this oil as a cure-all is not hyperbole. Tea tree essential oil can be used for a host of infections and diseases. The healing and disinfectant properties make it a wonder remedy that can boost immunity. However, it is absolutely not meant to be ingested because, used internally, it can turn to poison.[11] *Use topically only.* Tea tree essential oil is twelve times stronger than phenol, a common disinfectant used in hospitals.

Source

Tea tree essential oil is steam distilled from the leaves and twigs of the tea tree. Its scent has been described as astringent, acrid, camphorous, and medicinal, similar, but not identical, to eucalyptus.

Benefits

Tea tree essential oil is bactericide, antiviral, antifungal, antiseptic, expectorant, stimulant, and antimicrobial. Tea tree essential oil is known to be cleansing, purifying, uplifting and used externally for several conditions ranging from acne to athlete's foot, nail fungus, infections, wounds, lice abatement,

---

11. Soloway, Rose Ann Gould, *National Capital Poison Center.* Accessed Jan 15, 2019. https://www.poison.org/articles/2010-dec/tea-tree-oil.

for oral candidiasis (thrush), external cold sores, dandruff, and as a relief for skin lesions.

Tea tree is a very safe essential oil that possesses a strong camphorous, balsamic, and pungent odor emanating from the crushed plant leaves. Because it has potent and effective antibacterial, antifungal, and antiviral properties, it is a *must* for a home healing kit. Tea tree essential oil is best used externally unless you work with a trained Aromatherapist.

Precautions

Diluted tea tree essential oil is probably safe for most people when put on the skin, but it can cause skin irritation and swelling. When used for acne, it can sometimes cause skin dryness, itching, stinging, burning, and redness. Do a patch test on your skin to determine sensitivity. Be sure to keep out of your eyes when applying to the face. You may experience redness and irritation if you use too close to the delicate eye tissue. Despite the widespread claims that you can use this neat, undiluted, don't take the chance. You could end up with a red spot, a blister, or worse. Essential oils are powerful and potent.

Creative Ways to Use Tea Tree (*Melaleuca alternifolia*) Essential Oil

- Apply two to three drops of diluted tea tree essential oil to soothe minor burns. It can also help prevent scars from forming.

- A drop or two of diluted tea tree essential oil applied to the face as a bacterial wash will help breakouts and blemished skin. One diluted dab on acne can reduce redness and swelling.

- For a refreshing massage, dilute ten drops of tea tree essential oil in one ounce of carrier oil and massage over the body for tension and stress relief.

- Added to your mouthwash, a few drops of tea tree essential oil can help alleviate mouth infection or inflamed gums. (Avoid swallowing!)

- Eczema and dermatitis respond well to a mix of several drops of tea tree essential oil with a pure carrier oil and applied to the affected area. Carrier oils to use include borage, evening primrose, flaxseed, or kukui nut.

- Add tea tree essential oil to bathwater to treat bronchial congestion, hacking cough, and pulmonary inflammation. Use a proper dispersant.

- Congestion can be alleviated by rubbing a drop of diluted tea tree essential oil between your palms and inhaling deeply.

- Diluted tea tree essential oil is effective for persistent coughs when used in inhalers and diffusers.

- Diffuse a few drops of tea tree essential oil to ease chest congestion. Add four drops of tea tree essential oil to an open pan of boiling water properly dispersed, cover your head with a towel, close your eyes, and inhale the steam to alleviate congestion, colds, and coughs. (Don't bend too close to the steaming pan to avoid burns.)

- Head lice can be destroyed by adding a small amount of tea tree essential oil to shampoo.

- Freshen up your fabrics by using a spray bottle mixed with two cups of water and two teaspoons of tea tree essential oil. Test the fabric for staining before spraying the stale-smelling area. Let it rest for a few days. Most of the musty scent and the pungent tea tree essential oil smell will dissipate.

- Create an all-purpose cleaner by adding to two cups of water and two teaspoons of tea tree essential oil in a clean spray bottle. Shake well before using each time. This same mixture will also control mold.

- For sanitized and germ-free dishes and glasses, add a few drops of tea tree essential oil to your dishwasher dispenser. Then fill with a biodegradable dishwashing soap.

- Adding a few drops of tea tree essential oil to your laundry leaves your clothes smelling cleaner and helps to keep the storage bugs away.

- To repel insects, add ten to twenty drops of tea tree essential oil to two tablespoons of carrier oil and one tablespoon of aloe vera gel. Reapply every two to four hours.

- Use a tiny drop of diluted tea tree essential oil on blisters or insect bites.

Tea Tree *(Melaleuca alternifolia)*
Essential Oil Blends Nicely With

Clary sage, clove, rose geranium, lavender, lemon, rosemary, and thyme essential oils.

twenty-three

Thyme *(Thymus vulgaris)* Essential Oil

Thyme *(Thymus vulgaris)* is a perennial herb and member of the mint family. It has several outstanding healing properties due to the herb's powerful essential oils.

In Ancient Egypt, thyme was believed to help the dead crossover into the next life. Therefore, it was used in funeral preparation and embalming. The Greeks also liked it and burned thyme outside their temples to purify the space. The word thyme is thought to come from the Greek word *thumos,* meaning *smoke,* because of temple purification rituals. The Greeks also burned the herb before games and physical contests because it was thought to invoke courage. Virgil, the Roman poet, cited it as a cure for exhaustion.

Many Roman emperors drank a drop of thyme essential oil before feasting just in case some enemy doctored his wine or meal, as they believed it was an antidote to poison.

Thyme was a visible badge of honor in the Middle Ages. Knights setting off to battle wore sprigs of it on their armor for courage and protection.

Thyme has many magical attributes. Victorians believed a patch of thyme found in the woods signified the presence of faeries. It has been called the superstar of a garden. Young women during the Middle Ages were encouraged to sleep with thyme under their pillows so they would dream of the man they would marry.

I love thyme. I have grown my own cooking herbs for decades and thyme is a very satisfying herb to grow. From it I have made some savory dinners as well as some very wonderful tinctures, salves, and balms. Now I use the essential oil in massages and when I need a lift. It's so useful around the house, I probably use it at least once or twice a week without blinking. I think you'll come to treasure it, too.

Source

Thyme essential oil is steam distilled from the fresh flowers and leaves of the *Thymus vulgaris* plant. Thyme's fragrance is as a very powerful herb, pungent and slightly bitter, but its taste (the herb in food) is gentle, earthy, and lemony.

Benefits

Thyme essential oil is powerful. It has properties that are antibacterial, antiviral, a stimulant, antispasmodic, parasiticidal, and expectorant.

It is used to relieve and treat problems like gout, arthritis, wounds, bites, sores, water retention, menstrual and menopausal problems, nausea and fatigue, respiratory problems (colds), skin conditions (oily skin and scars), athlete's foot, hangovers, and even depression by diffusing or inhaling the strong scent of thyme essential oil. I tend to think of it as an essential oil that's a real tough guy or gal: the Annie Oakley of the essential oil set.

The Technological Educational Institute of Ionian Islands, Greece, tested the antimicrobial activity of eight plant essential oils in 2010. Their research concluded that thyme essential oil was the best at eliminating bacteria from the test petri dish within sixty minutes. Very impressive results![12]

Among the essential oils tested in another study, cinnamon essential oil and thyme essential oil were found to be the most successful destroyers of Staphylococcus bacteria, including the dreaded MRSA.[13]

The benefits of thyme essential oil have been recognized for thousands of years in Mediterranean countries. The wise ones knew it had antibacterial qualities, so it was used in drinks, soups, stews, breads, as well as in medicinal salves and tonics. We refer to the chemotype "thyme ct. Linalool" as our thyme essential oil of choice.

---

12. *WorldWideScience.org,* accessed Feb 2, 2019. https://worldwidescience. org/topicpages/p/plant+essential+oil.html.
13. Ibid.

Precautions

Thyme essential oil should not be used directly on skin, as it can cause an allergic reaction. Thyme essential oil is not recommended for people with hyperthyroidism, as it may overstimulate the thyroid gland.

Thyme essential oil can increase circulation; therefore, it should be avoided by people with high blood pressure. Pregnant women should avoid thyme essential oil because it can stimulate menstrual flow. Due to its strength, thyme essential oil should not be used on infants and young children.

Creative Ways to Use Thyme (*Thymus vulgaris*) Essential Oil

- Diffuse thyme essential oil to stimulate the mind, strengthen the memory, improve concentration, and calm the nerves.

- Use thyme essential oil as a treatment to stimulate the scalp and prevent hair loss by adding a few drops to shampoo and other hair products. Mix only what you will use per application. Do not let the essential oil sit in the bottle with the shampoo or conditioner.

- Thyme essential oil can help tone aged skin and prevent acne outbreaks. Dilute in a carrier oil before applying topically and avoid the eye area.

- Thyme essential oil can be used to fight bad breath and reduce gum inflammation. Add a few drops to your mouthwash: two drops per one teaspoon of mouthwash. Do not swallow.

- A few drops of thyme essential oil can keep insects and parasites like mosquitoes, fleas, lice, and moths away. Dilute two drops in one teaspoon of a carrier oil before rubbing directly onto skin as a repellant.

- For pain relief, mix three drops of thyme essential oil with two teaspoons of sesame oil. Use this mixture as a massage oil and apply on the abdominal area to relieve pain. Always massage abdominal area in a clockwise motion.

- The same mixture of thyme essential oil above can be used as a massage oil to treat other types of pain as well.

- To alleviate fatigue, add two drops of thyme essential oil to your bathwater diluted in a proper dispersant.

- For restful sleep, add a few drops to your diffuser.

- To reduce the appearance of scars and skin marks, apply thyme essential oil mixed with a carrier oil (like borage or apricot kernel) on the affected area.

- For a facial and skin cleanser, mix a few drops of thyme essential oil into your facial wash product.

- To use as a treatment for, or to protect against, respiratory problems, add two drops of thyme essential oil properly dispersed to hot water and use for steam inhalation.

- To uplift a sad mood, add two drops of thyme essential oil to a dampened cloth, cotton ball, or handkerchief and inhale the revitalizing scent.

Thyme *(Thymus vulgaris)*
Essential Oil Blends Nicely With

Lavender, lemon, orange, rosemary, and pine essential oils.

twenty-four

Ylang-Ylang *(Cananga odorata)* Essential Oil

Ylang-ylang is the Malay name for *flower of flowers.* It comes from a small tropical tree native to the Philippines. Cultivated trees provide the floral, heady, sweet aroma of ylang-ylang, whereas wild ones do not provide the same desirable, intense scent. In Asia, the flowers have long been valued for their aphrodisiac fragrance, which was originally extracted by maceration in coconut oil.

Because ylang-ylang essential oil has a powerful and uplifting, recognizable aroma, it is sometimes called Cheap Man's Jasmine. Ylang-ylang trees are visible along the roadside throughout Malaysia where it is planted to provide shade by day and a beautiful scent in the night air. It is also used for decoration at festivals and celebrations combined with jasmine, rose, and the very sought-after champaca.

Ylang-ylang essential oil is frequently used as an ingredient in aphrodisiac incense blends. The flowers of the ylang-ylang are traditionally spread on the wedding bed in southeast Asia for extra special sensuous arousal because the scent is reputed to relax and calm wedding night fears and anxieties.

Ylang-ylang essential oil brings our emotional and sensual natures together if they have drifted apart. Ylang-ylang is a soul-centering essential oil that unites the heart and the mind to soothe, open, and harmonize the whole body. Doesn't that sound dreamy?

This floral essential oil is among my top favorites. I use a lava bead bracelet to soak up a diluted dose of ylang-ylang essential oil. I wear the bracelet so the aroma of the intoxicating ylang-ylang blossoms remains with me throughout the day. It lasts from the first breakfast meeting through the evening yoga class. It retains its fragrance even when I drive home after stretching and relieving the tensions of the workday. Many a day it has brought me calm in the face of would-be anxiety and taken the edge off several crispy encounters.

Ylang-ylang essential oil has the feel of ancient rites and ceremonies. It brings me in touch with the wisdom of the past. I feel like I am not alone on this planet when I wear something infused with ylang-ylang. It has been my friend through many emotional crises. I hope you will claim it as your friend, too. When it comes to essential oil friends, we can't ever have enough, and we don't have to text them or remember their birthdays. They are easy friends to have.

Source

The flowers of the cananga odorata tree are steam distilled for extraction of the ylang-ylang essential oil. Ylang-ylang essential oil is beautifully fragrant, with a heavy, sweet, slightly fruity, floral scent. It is the main note in the famous Chanel N°5 perfume.

Benefits

Ylang-ylang boasts the properties of being an antidepressant, aphrodisiac, antiseptic, antispasmodic, anti-inflammatory, and antiparasitic. French chemists, Garnier and Rechler, recognized ylang-ylang's medicinal properties at the beginning of the twentieth century during their research on Réunion Island where they found it to be effective against malaria, typhus, and infections of the intestinal tract, as well as having a calming effect on the heart.

Ylang-ylang essential oil is primarily used for its positive psychological properties and helping people to overcome negativity, fears, inhibitions, feelings of low self-worth, self-hatred, inferiority, and insecurity. Ylang-ylang essential oil therapy provides emotional clearing, insomnia relief, dispels negativity, alleviates jealousy, and reduces anger and fever. It combats low self-esteem and restores confidence. Also, ylang-ylang essential oil is appreciated for its ability to help regulate cardiac arrhythmia, forestall hair loss, and neutralize intestinal problems.

Ylang-ylang essential oil is used for soothing insect stings and bites, as well as general skin care. It's used as a body rub to prevent fever and infections as well as nourishing and rejuvenating the skin.

Precautions

Avoid ylang-ylang essential oil in the first trimester of pregnancy. Avoid using on inflamed skin or skin affected by dermatitis. Excessive use of ylang-ylang can cause headaches and nausea.

Creative Ways to Use Ylang-Ylang (*Cananga odorata*) Essential Oil

- When diffused, ylang-ylang essential oil can be effective for helping chest infections, bronchitis, and spasmodic coughs.

- Ylang-ylang essential oil can be used on different types of skin, including sensitive and oily as well as dry and mature due to its skin-renewing and moisture-retention properties. Add a few drops of ylang-ylang essential oil to your favorite body cream or facial tonic for softer and rejuvenated skin.

- Ylang-ylang essential oil is nourishing and moisturizing for dry, dehydrated, or irritated skin.

- For split ends, add several drops of ylang-ylang essential oil to your favorite shampoo or conditioner.

- Make a miracle moisturizing hair treatment by using four to six drops of ylang-ylang essential oil mixed with one to two teaspoons of coconut or jojoba oil. Massage into hair, place a shower cap on your head, and allow this to permeate your hair overnight. It's also good for hair growth.

- To relieve PMS or menopause symptoms, combine three drops of ylang-ylang essential oil with one drop each of bergamot, sandalwood, geranium, and lavender essential oils for a diffuser blend. Use the same mixture diluted in a carrier oil for a clockwise massage of the pelvic area. Avoid using on genitals.

- Add a few drops of ylang-ylang essential oil to your bath for relaxation. Use a proper dispersant. (See chapter 4.)

- For circulatory system health, mix two to three drops of ylang-ylang essential oil in one ounce of carrier oil and massage on the body.

- To release anger or frustration, diffuse one drop of ylang-ylang essential oil with two drops of frankincense essential oil.

- For a super sexy night, diffuse eight drops ylang-ylang essential oil with six drops of sandalwood essential oil and nine drops of orange essential oil in your bedroom diffuser. Dim the lights, add some romantic music, and write me a thank you note the next morning.

- For a calm and peaceful feeling, diffuse three drops of ylang-ylang essential oil with three drops of lavender and four drops of Roman chamomile essential oils.

- To promote healthy self-esteem, blend two drops of ylang-ylang essential oil with one drop of bergamot essential oil. Diffuse or mix with a carrier oil to use as a massage oil.

Ylang-Ylang *(Cananga odorata)* Essential Oil Blends Nicely With

Patchouli, lavender, bergamot, rose, frankincense, clove bud, lemon, and orange essential oils.

There you have it. An overview of twenty essential oils that can give you instant first aid medication, longer-term skin and hair improvement, cosmetic and wrinkle assistance, monthly pain relief, overall chronic and temporary aches and pain relief, and some preventative measures to stave off illness and aging. So, how are you feeling about these twenty essential oils? Do they appeal to you so far? Are you ready to try a few and see how they can improve your life?

I know it's a lot to take in, and my beginning students are usually raring to go at this point in the lessons and want to move on to putting these amazing essential oils to use. After thirty some years with essential oils, I still learn new things every time I read or research an essential oil. I am still learning. If you are new to the world of essential oils, my advice is to pick out a few of your favorites. Get to know them, use them, experiment with them, and, after some experience with a few basic starting oils, branch out from there. If you master a few essential oils first, you will have better results long term. The first ones end up being our greatest teachers.

In part 3 we will learn about the differences and notes of the different essential oils, how to blend them, and how to use them in diffusers for multiple conditions, for the mind and emotions, and for spiritual and ritual purposes. We're ready to move into the real fun and excitement of working with essential oils.

part 3

Putting Essential Oils to Use

Without a doubt, this is the portion you've been waiting for. It's the time when you can put all this knowledge to work and begin to make some wonderful blends and scrumptious products for yourself, your friends, and family.

In the next section you'll learn some tips that the most experienced perfumers in Paris use for making their legendary scents. Then you can put your fresh knowledge to use and begin making your own signature scents.

Your world expands even more into personal products you can make and use every day. With this knowledge you'll be able to save a bundle on expensive over-the-counter creams, lotions, and spa products. You will have the keys to beauty creams and therapeutic balms that will serve you during all four seasons of hot and cold weather.

The section you might find the most useful for everyday aches and pains is chapter 28, which features essential oil recommendations for seventy-six common complaints that can be abated by using the suggestions contained in this A–Z listing.

We end this section with more blends that can help you deal with the everyday challenges of anxiety, stress, exhaustion, irritability, and mental fatigue. Finally, we'll end on a spiritual note with some ideas for interesting and meaningful ways you can use essential oils to enrich your life and the lives of those closest to you.

If you're ready, let's move ahead into the world of possibilities with essential oils.

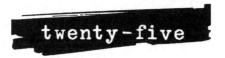

Insider Tips on Blending
Essential Oils

We've come a long way on our journey with essential oils. I hope you've already purchased and experimented with some of your new essential oils by now. If you're ready to kick it up a notch and try some creative blending magic of your own, let's get started.

One of the best things you can learn about essential oils is how they go together. You can experiment on your own and learn through trial and error, but what I'm about to share with you can help you take a shortcut to successful blends and the secrets the best perfumer creators in the world use to achieve perfection when they create the scents of legends.

These guidelines are helpful to keep in mind as you start becoming an expert blender.

There are companies that manufacture blends claiming to bring you harmony, peace, and relief of this or that condition or ailment. I recommend you blend your own because that gives you complete control of the quality and properties of the essential oils that go into your blend.

The Three Notes: Top, Middle, and Base

If you create a fragrance blend, you will want to add a Top note, a Middle note, and a Base note for balance.

There is a lot of advice available on the internet about which oils to blend together and how to blend them according to the category of notes that the essential oil falls into. The categories were assessed, classified, and recorded by George William Septimus Piesse in his book, *The Art of Perfumery*. He also created a device known as the *odaphone*, which utilized a scent scale to rank the odor of perfumes.

The first time I heard about notes for essential oils, I thought I was in a music class by mistake. As I became more familiar with the different notes of the essential oils, I realized it was a virtual symphony of aromas and moods I could create using the guideline. This information gave me the freedom to become the maestro of my own aromatic symphony.

According to the odaphone scale, there are three note categories an essential oil can fall into: Top, Middle, or Base. Balancing notes can make the scent linger longer.

Top Notes

Essential oils that are classified as Top notes normally evaporate very fast. They are fast-acting and usually give the bold first impression of the blend you make.

Top note essential oils include: bergamot, clary sage, eucalyptus, lemon, orange, peppermint, tea tree, and thyme

Middle Notes

These essential oils give body to the blend and are the *balancers*. The Middle notes may not be immediately evident and may take a few minutes to be recognized, but they are the core of the blend. They are usually warm and soft smelling.

Middle note essential oils include: Roman chamomile, geranium, lavender, Melissa, pine, rose, and rosemary

Base Notes

They are normally heavy oils and their fragrance is quite evident and forward, but they can also slowly evolve and are potent for a longer time. They also slow the evaporation of the other oils. They are heady and intense-smelling and many can be costly. But they are worth their weight in gold because they sustain the fragrance of the blend.

Base note essential oils include: clove, frankincense, patchouli, sandalwood, and ylang-ylang

Additional Methods for Categorizing

You can group essential oils by a couple of different scales: by purpose or scent group.

Purpose

Energizing: bergamot, clary sage, clove, eucalyptus, lemon, peppermint, pine, rosemary, tea tree

Calming: bergamot, geranium, lavender, Melissa, orange, patchouli, rose, sandalwood, ylang-ylang

Detoxing: eucalyptus, lemon, patchouli, peppermint, rosemary, tea tree, thyme

Relaxing: bergamot, frankincense, geranium, lavender, Melissa, Roman chamomile, rose, sandalwood

Toning: geranium, rose

Uplifting: lemon, Melissa, orange, pine

Scent Group

Citrus: bergamot, lemon, orange

Earthy: frankincense, patchouli, sandalwood

Floral: geranium, lavender, rose, ylang-ylang

Herby: clary sage, thyme

Medicinal: eucalyptus, rosemary, tea tree

Minty: peppermint

Oriental: patchouli

Spicy: clove

Woodsy: pine

I've listed categories for you because essential oils from the same category will blend well together. Essential oils in one category can also be matched and blended with oils in compatible categories. Citrus goes well with spicy; citrus goes well with floral; woodsy works well with floral; and herbal and citrus make great aromatic friends.

Only you can determine what your specific needs are and only you can assess how your body responds to the various essential oils. Select the correct essential oil for the purpose you intend.

Try It Yourself: Creating a Blend

Blending essential oils is all about inhaling, experimentation, and creating fragrances that suit you. It is one of the most creative and intuitive uses for essential oils. Blending requires preparation and time, but the end product is worth it. These guidelines are helpful to keep in mind as you start becoming an expert blender.

Always use sterile conditions. Don't blend in the sun, and allow enough time to combine and rest the essential oil blend before diluting or using them. The oils need time to become friends and share their chemical components to create the aroma you want.

Try to limit your blend to three or four essential oils for your first session. Take into consideration the purpose of the blend. What are you trying to accomplish? Is it a blend for a diffuser, an inhaler, for massage, or for direct application to clear up a condition? Are you working on the physical, emotional, or spiritual level? Is this for yourself or another person? Purpose is very important. Also, be sure to follow all safety guidelines and check the contraindications for each essential oil prior to using them in your blends, perfumes, and recipes.

Supplies you will need

- Several 3 x 5 cards or a journal to take notes so you will know how to remake a successful formula
- Labels for your bottles (top or side)

- A pen or felt-tip marker
- A few 15-ml dark glass bottles
- Essential oils
- Carrier oils
- Mixing bottles (small 2-ml amber or blue glass)
- Perfume testing strips
- Protective latex or non-latex gloves
- Pipettes
- Paper towels
- Extra carrier oil to clean up spills

When you begin blending, start small. You can always increase the quantity later when you decide you like a scent or blend you create. Here are the steps to follow.

Step One: Consider Aroma

What aromas do you like? Herby, floral, spicy, foresty? Decide on what you want to end up with before you begin. Select the essential oils you want to use. Starting small means to pick a blend that will take five, ten, twenty, or twenty-five drops in order to waste less. You'll be mixing your blends in small bottles, so have your tools and ingredients handy.

Step Two: The Sniff Test

Perform a sniff test on the essential oils you have chosen to work with. Place one drop of each on your perfume test strips. Label the bottom of the strip with the essential oil you used. Draw the strip up to your nose after waving it in circles around you twelve inches away from your body. How does it smell when you are a foot away? Determine the distance you can still smell the aroma. Is it two feet, three feet, four feet, six feet, or more?

Step Three: Keep a Record

Take notes. Using a journal or the 3 x 5 cards, notate the distance from which you can smell the aroma. Record your impressions of the aroma, how it makes you feel, and whether it is pronounced or faint. What category does it fit into? Is this a sharp or dull scent? Is it heavy or light? Repeat these steps for every essential oil you want to use in your blend. Take notes and then place all of them in your hand, creating an aroma wand to circle around in the air. What do you smell now that they are together? Remove the strips of those that you have chosen not to work with. Set everything down and take a short break for fifteen to thirty minutes.

Step Four: Repeat the Sniff Test

Return to your work area and repeat the sniff test of the selected strips. How did they hold up after some time? Are they still potent and active? Have some dissipated? How do they make you feel? How do they make your body feel? After you record your notes, select the strips that you want to blend and categorize them into Top, Middle, or Base notes.

Step Five: Create Your Blend

Now you will create your blend. Using the 2-ml bottles, work with the percentages of:

Top note—30 percent, Middle note—50 percent, and Base note—20 percent. Begin with one drop. Add two drops, then add a fourth. When you have made your blend, shake it around to blend it and add one drop of it to a perfume test strip. Wave it in the air again and inhale the aroma. How did you do? Is this the one? Do you need to add any more of one or two of the oils? Repeat the process until you have the blend you like. Does it suit your purpose?

Step Six: Using Your Blend

At this point, you will decide what you are going to do with the blend. Will you diffuse it? Will you dilute it with other essential oils or carrier oils to make another product? Will you try your hand at making a perfume or a cologne?

If you are going to save the blend for dermal application, use a 15-ml dark glass bottle and pour the mixture into the new bottle. Make sure you only have eight drops of essential oil mixture in the bottle for this 15-ml size. Add a carrier oil such as sweet almond, jojoba, or an oil of your choice that fits a specific purpose (e.g., skin, wounds, wrinkles, etc.). Be careful to note if you have used phototoxic oils in your mix, as this will affect how you use the blend.

Blend Recipes for Scenting Your Body

Instead of using over-the-counter fragrances that can be filled with chemicals and toxins, you can make your own signature scents by following the recipes below. It's simple, but it will take a few weeks to cure, so you want to avoid making it on Friday for your Saturday-night date. The curing process is essential because this is the time it takes for the essential oil molecules to marry and comingle their aromas. Shake the bottle once a day to stimulate the molecules as they meld together to create the fragrance.

Signature Scent

- 7–15 drops of the blend of your choice
- 1 Tbsp. jojoba or sweet almond oil (215 drops)

Mix together and keep in a 15-ml dark glass bottle. Do not diffuse this blend. Use this blend for scenting your body or diluted in a massage blend.

Perfume

- 4 tsp. of 190-proof vodka, Everclear, or pharmaceutical-grade 200-proof alcohol
- 1¼ tsp. of distilled water (add this after curing)
- 1 tsp. carrier oil like sweet almond or jojoba
- 28 drops of your *Signature Scent* blend

Store in an airtight container for ten to fourteen days. Open and strain through a coffee filter or laboratory-grade filter paper. Add distilled water. Re-bottle, in the same bottle if you choose, and allow to cure for three more weeks. You can decant this into a perfume atomizer or bottle after it has cured.

Cologne

- 4½ tsp. of 190-proof vodka, Everclear, or pharmaceutical-grade grain alcohol
- 2 tsp. distilled water (add after curing)
- ½ tsp. carrier oil
- 20 drops of essential oils

Store in an airtight container for ten to fourteen days. Open and strain through a coffee filter or laboratory-grade filter paper. Add distilled water. Re-bottle, in the same bottle if you choose, and allow to cure for two more weeks. Decant into a bottle of your choice thereafter.

Blend Recipes for Inhalers, Roll-Ons, and Hand Sanitizers

There are other things you can make using your blending skills like inhalers, roll-ons, and hand sanitizers. The inhalers we discuss here are the portable inhalers you use for colds and not the prescription inhalers and bronchodilators for conditions like asthma or COPD. The inhalers are blanks and come in kits and can be found online or in health food stores where essential oils are sold.

The Germ-Preventing Inhaler

It's a handy way to carry around a mini-pharmacy in a tube. Inhalers are excellent for travel and they can be created for antibiotic reasons, pleasant aromas, as a decongestant, or as a pure source of relaxation and tranquility. You can design your own center of calm by using lavender or you can create an energy source with lemon and peppermint. I like to think of inhalers as Quick Fix Sticks.

Supplies you will need
- Several 3" x 5" cards or a journal to take notes so you will know how to remake a successful formula
- Some labels
- A pen or felt-tip marker
- A few inhaler or inhaler kits, which you can buy online

- Wicks (organic cotton, not bleached or chemically treated). These are in addition to the ones that may come with inexpensive inhaler kits. Opt for organic and unbleached for your safety.
- Essential oils
- Carrier oils
- Mixing containers (small 2" x 2")
- Plastic spoons or clean Popsicle sticks to stir with
- Protective latex or non-latex gloves
- Tweezers
- Paper towels
- Essential oils: eucalyptus, peppermint, rosemary, tea tree, orange, lemon
- Extra carrier oil to clean up spills.

Directions

1. Take the bottom off the inhaler and unscrew the top part. Remove the wick from the inhaler and set aside. If your inhaler comes with a cheap wick, throw it away and use the unbleached cotton ones you purchased separately.

2. In a small container, combine the essential oils: five drops of eucalyptus, two drops of peppermint, two drops of rosemary, two drops of tea tree, three drops of orange, two drops of lemon, and one teaspoon of carrier oil.

3. Mix the essential oils well. Drop the wick into the container with the essential oil blends and roll it around using a clean spoon or Popsicle stick. Allow

the mixture to sit until the wick has absorbed all, or most of, the oils. (If you are using a plastic container, the essential oils can melt the plastic if left in the container for more than a few hours.)

4. Using your tweezers, pick up the oil-saturated wick and place it into the inhaler tube. Snap the bottom back on and voilà, you have a fantastic inhaler that will help you ward off seasonal germs and keep you breathing clearly all year long. This inhaler will most likely last you sixty to ninety days before you need to refresh it.

I keep my little container with a snap-on lid, label it with the ingredients I used, and put it away for next time. I store this in a cool, dark place so the oils don't go bad. If you leave it too long, wash it out and start fresh.

The Relaxation Rollerball

You can make your own rollerball in much the same way. Let's make one with a formula for your feet to generate relaxation from a busy day.

Supplies you will need

- An empty 15-ml rollerball (buy the dark ones to keep damaging light rays out: blue, amber, or amethyst)
- A rolling ball top (usually comes with the rollerball kit)
- Pipettes to control the amount of carrier oil and essential oils put into the bottle (use one pipette per essential oil)
- Gloves for protection

- Essential oils: eucalyptus, rosemary, lavender, lemon, ylang-ylang
- Carrier oil like rose hip or sweet almond

Directions

1. Unscrew the cap of the rollerball bottle and set aside.
2. Remove the rollerball plug.
3. Using individual pipettes, add twelve drops of eucalyptus, ten drops of rosemary, ten drops of lavender, two drops of lemon, and five drops of ylang-ylang to the empty rollerball bottle.
4. Fill the bottle up with the carrier oil using a pipette, leaving enough room to replace the plug. Put the cap back on, label the rollerball with the ingredients, shake it well to blend, and you're ready to roll.
5. You can use this blend on your feet, or you can also roll it around the back of your neck and temples for relaxation.
6. It's a good idea to get into bed first before using the roller on the bottoms of your feet. The oils are slippery, so you don't want to grease up your feet and go for a stroll. Also, the oils could mark your flooring and carpets. Once you use essential oils on your feet, remain prone until they absorb.

The AWEsome Day Rollerball

The formula for my AWEsome Day rollerball is:

1. Follow the instructions above. Add to the empty 15-ml empty rollerball bottle ten drops of lavender, ten drops of orange, and five drops of peppermint.

2. Fill the bottle with carrier oil and shake well to blend.

3. Replace the rolling ball and the cap, label it, and off you go on your AWEsome Day.

Hand Sanitizer, Sparkle

Supplies you will need

- Hand sanitizer bottle or dispenser. (Use the empty containers when the store-bought product has been used or purchase empty containers, which can be found in stores and online.)
- 3 pipettes
- 1 oz. aloe vera gel (or 2 oz. if you buy a larger container)
- 8 drops lavender, 5 drops orange, 2 drops lemon

Directions

1. Mix all ingredients well.

2. Label it.

3. Carry with you and use when needed.
   The aloe vera gel will make your hands soft and supple and, by making your own, you know you're using ingredients that are good for you and that you control.

———

Are you getting excited about all the wonderful items you can make in your own kitchen? I hope so. The beauty of making your own products is that after an initial set up, the costs go down and this becomes a sustainable hobby. You're working with natural products, and for every single one you make you are contributing toward a healthier and more ecologically balanced world.

Next, we're going to learn all about diffusers and which ones will work the best for you and your needs. It's a thorough compendium of information that will make your shopping easier and point to which one(s) will work best for your lifestyle.

twenty-six

Inhalation—All About Diffusers and Diffusing

D iffusers are a subject that always comes up in my classes. Students want to know which ones are the best, the safest, and the easiest to maintain. There are so many brands in the marketplace that it would take a full edition of *Consumer Reports* to analyze them all.

People love diffusers because they create an invisible aroma that can be enjoyable as well as healing. Essential oils diffused into the air can keep germs at bay, cleanse the air of harmful bacteria, ward off insects, improve breathing, break up chest congestion, improve and enhance mental capacity, induce sleep, relieve pain, deepen your meditation practice, boost energy, reduce food cravings, and more.

Types of Diffusers

There are many types of diffusers available. The ones I recommend are ultrasonic, evaporation, nebulizer, room sprays, reed diffusers, travel diffusers, and jewelry. There are also heat diffusers, oil burners, candles, or electric lamps, but I do not recommend these, and we'll get into why with each item.

Ultrasonic

Water and essential oils are dispersed as fine mists into the environment through vibrations. They don't use heat, so the integrity of the essential oil is maintained. A central, ceramic diaphragm vibrates at a high frequency, which transforms the diffuser's water supply combined with the essential oil droplets into a mist. This device also works as a room humidifier when essential oils are not added to the water. Either way, this fine mist enters the body when it's breathed into the lungs.

Some diffusers can run for ten consecutive hours. Others run for 30 to 120 minutes. With all ultrasonic diffusers, you have to remember to give it a good cleaning whenever it needs it so it can continue to work smoothly and healthily for you. Ultrasonic devices come in a wide variety of materials, including glass, bamboo, stone, ceramic, wood, and plastic.

For best results use distilled water in this diffuser with your essential oils. Only a few drops of essential oil are required. These diffusers will add humidity to the room, so make sure that's a side effect you want and need.

If you live in a space with mold or mildew, do not use the ultrasonic diffuser until you clear up the condition. Ultrasonic diffusers add moisture to the room, so that is not what you want to bring to this situation.

Check the viscosity and thickness of the essential oils before you use them in a diffuser. Be wary of frankincense, myrrh, benzoin, vetiver, patchouli, and elemi. Only use essential oils that are thin, or you will clog your device and render it useless. If an essential oil is hard to get out of the bottle or comes out slowly, that's an indication you should not use it in your diffuser.

Limit your selection to two or three essential oils in the diffuser. More than two or three oils can overwhelm the senses and cause headaches and sensitization if it's too potent a mix.

Because of the dilution of essential oils in the water, the therapeutic effects are not as pronounced as *nebulizers* (see description below), which do not use water.

Begin to acclimate your senses to the essential-oil-scented air. Start with fifteen minutes per day and work your way up to a longer amount of time. Do not overwhelm your senses, nasal passages, or sensitive olfactory tissue by using diffused essential oils for more than an hour at a time.

Evaporation

An internal fan blows the essential oil scents into the air through a pad or a filter. Essential oils are dropped onto an internal felt pad and the central fan sends it out into the atmosphere.

Nebulizer

The main difference between a diffuser and a nebulizer is a diffuser uses evaporated water particles to carry the essential oil out into the air, whereas a nebulizer breaks down the molecules of the essential oil, atomizes them, and turns them into a gaseous state before sending the gasses into the room. This is a positive thing. A nebulizer transforms an essential oil into molecules and releases them into the air without using water molecules.

To use a nebulizer, pour a 10-ml bottle of your chosen essential oil, or 10-ml of a blend of essential oils, directly into the diffuser for powerful, continuous diffusion. The unit uses no heat or water. An air pump breaks apart the molecules of the essential oils and releases them into the air in the form of tiny droplets, creating a fine mist or spray. Nebulization allows the full advantage use of the active therapeutic principles of essentials oils.

Be cautious of very resinous oils like frankincense, sandalwood, patchouli, and possibly pine. If they are too thick to be properly diffused or nebulized, they can harm your machine.

You never want to put carrier oils in your nebulizer because they are thicker and cannot atomize and will, therefore, clog your nebulizer. You will waste your essential oils and carrier oils. One thing to be aware of is that nebulizers produce a buzzing sound, so they are not the quietest version of diffusers. But they can be very effective if you don't mind a soft buzzing.

Nebulizers also can consume a lot of essential oils. The good news is that it is advisable to only run them for ten to fifteen minutes at a time. Some units come equipped with pulse timers you can program for the short releases and wait times in between. These can be costly to run even though they are wonderfully effective. It depends on how expensive your essential oils are and your personal budget. Personally, I believe they're worth it.

Room Sprays

Sprays are a nice way to freshen a room. Fill a four-ounce spray bottle with witch hazel, which adds another level of antibacterial quality to the spray, and add nine drops of essential oil for each ounce of liquid in the sprayer. This is a 1 percent dilution. Eighteen drops per ounce makes it a 2 percent dilution. You can use plain water, but you need to add a preservative to the mixture, like 160–190 proof vodka (two teaspoons) or Optiphen Plus. The preservative extends the life of your product beyond one month and keeps the water free from bacteria, germs, yeast, and mold. If you use it within thirty days, you can skip the preservatives. Be sure to shake the mixture each time before you spray. Get in the habit of shaking your concoctions with essential oils well to make sure the oils have not separated from the rest of the ingredients.

You can make room sprays for different rooms in the house by using scents suitable for each room. Lemon or orange are great for bathrooms, lavender and eucalyptus or rosemary for the living room, ylang-ylang and geranium for the bedroom, and lemon or orange for the kitchen.

Reed Diffusers

These are another wonderful way to gently and consistently fill a room with a selected essential oil's aroma. Think of it like a flower arrangement that continually permeates the air with its scent. The beauty of making your own reed diffuser is that you can get as creative and unique as you want to. There are many bottles you can choose from that fit your style and décor.

It is best to make your own reed diffusers. The ones you buy commercially are filled with adulterated oils that can cause hormone disruption and other undesirable outcomes. Many contain 70 percent isopropyl alcohol (rubbing alcohol), which can be deadly if consumed. Children can get ahold of these reed diffusers if they are left within reach in bathrooms, boudoirs, or living spaces. Bottom line: make your own and choose a safe place for it. Here are the directions:

DIY Reed Diffuser

Items you will need include:

- A glass jar or vase with a narrow opening at the top (check your local thrift stores)
- 6–8 rattan diffuser reeds (available online, buy a couple dozen)
- ¼ to ½ cup carrier oil (jojoba and sweet almond are nice)
- ½–1 tsp. of witch hazel or pure vodka (use the highest proof you can find, 160–190 proof is optimal)
- 20–40 drops of essential oil of your choice

This is the time to use some of your older or nearing-expiration carrier oils. Make sure they are not cloudy, too viscous, or smell off. Use only carrier oils that are light in texture so they can easily make their way up the reeds.

This is also a great way to use some of your older or almost expired essential oils. Make sure they are not too far gone or have a rancid smell. Create blends of your favorites.

Directions

1. Clean your receptacle.
2. Add a light-textured carrier oil to the bottle. (Heavy oils will not travel up the reeds.)
3. Add the vodka or witch hazel as a thinner.
4. Add the essential oil drops or blends you have created.
5. Cover and gently shake the liquids to mix.

6. Add your rattan reeds.

7. Place in a safe area of the house and enjoy. The oils will saturate the reeds and fill the environment with their aroma.

You'll want to replenish your essential oils and carrier oil as they age or evaporate into the air. Be sure to keep the reed diffuser out of the reach of children and animals. When the reeds become overly saturated, you should replace them with fresh ones. Dispose of the reeds and oil mixture according to the proper disposal guidelines in chapter 3.

Portable Travel Diffusers

These little gems run on batteries, an electric cord, or sometimes plug into the USB port of a computer or laptop. Like reed diffusers, fan diffusers expose essential oils to air without heat. Drops of the essential oil are added to a pad inside, and the electric fan in the diffuser causes the oils on the pad to disperse into the air. This type of diffuser is extremely personal. It's good for use in the office, hotel rooms, and tight spaces. It fits in the palm of your hand and packs nicely. There are many versions available. Big box stores have affordable selections and brands.

The ones I like are Diffuse on the Move, Mini Portable Oil Diffuser, and Nature's Bounty Earthly Elements. The beautiful news is that big-box stores carry these items and you can have them shipped directly to your home or office. I have mixed feelings about the small diffusers that plug into your car or computer. They can be overwhelming and it's not safe to diffuse essential oils that might make you sleepy or drowsy when you drive. I don't think anyone wants to nod off in the middle of the fast lane.

It's a smart idea to have a portable diffuser for your hotel room or private office to keep the air clean and germ-free. I have a collection of three and I use them wherever I go. At home, I have diffusers in the bedroom, living room, and in my office. Each features a different blend of aromatics and I always ask visitors if they can tolerate essential oils before I switch the machine on.

The Old-Fashioned Method

Put a couple drops of carrier oil in your hands. Add the exact same number of drops of essential oil. Rub your hands together and make a tent over your nose with your hands, avoiding your eyes. Inhale. The aromas go directly into your brain. This is the most effective, potent, and inexpensive method you can use. If you want to heal something quickly, use this method.

Jewelry

Essential oils can be diffused by things you wear and infused with your choice of essential oils.

Pendant: There are many pendants you can buy that have felt pads inside. Soak the pads with your favorite scents and wear them all day. The pendant I wear is always soaked with peppermint and lemon essential oils. I use this for driving when I want to stay alert and when I teach classes or give workshops. They always give me a good boost so I can be as energetic at the end of the workshop as I was at the beginning. And, unlike caffeine, they don't wear off and leave me dragging.

Mine opens to reveal a felt pad. I add two to four drops of peppermint essential oil and a drop or two of lemon essential oil. It makes for a perky, crisp blend that lasts through a long drive or a four-hour workshop. The pendant needs to be refreshed once or twice a day.

Bracelet: There are also bracelet designs that have full or partial lava beads as part of the design. The lava beads are porous and absorb the essential oils, making them carriers of the aromas. The lava bracelet is my favorite choice for yoga, tai chi, and Qigong practices. I wear it when I exercise because the ylang-ylang or bergamot fragrance I choose keeps me centered in beauty and bliss. I love having the scents close by and they keep me focused on my practice. For some people they might "get in the way," but for me they work very well with the activity I am doing.

There are bracelets available that are strung with all lava beads, or you can find ones that have only a percentage of lava beads mixed with other stones. No matter which one you choose, it will be great. You can soak the lava bead bracelets in a mixture of essential oils diluted in a carrier oil and wear them all day to enjoy the scent they give off. The bracelet aroma usually lasts for a day or two. Do not soak anything other than the lava beads in this way. If you have a bracelet that is part lava bead and part other stones with silver or gold metal clasps or spacers, don't soak the bracelet. Instead, dilute a few drops of the essential oil of your choice and use a pipette to apply the mixture to the lava beads only. Allow the hybrid bracelet to hang or rest by itself on a piece of waxed paper, not a paper towel, for fifteen minutes before wearing.

If you have a full lava bead bracelet, find a little soaking container (a small bead container is great) and add four to six drops of a carrier oil to the container. Use lighter oils like jojoba or sweet almond. Drop three to four drops of your selected essential oil and stir together with a disposable wooden stick. Place the lava bead bracelet in the mixture and wait fifteen to twenty minutes. Move the bracelet around in the oil mixture to get all the beads covered.

Some people will advise you to drop the essential oils directly onto the beads, neat. You don't want to do that. It means putting the full-strength essential oils next to your skin. Be sure you dilute the essential oils before you soak your bracelet or beads to avoid skin irritation. I can tell you from my direct experience that using the oil neat is not a good idea.

Heat Diffusion (Not recommended)

The energy of heat disperses essential oils into the air. One drawback is that high heat is not as effective as low heat in the distribution of essential oils. Higher heat can destroy the essential oil's chemistry and, in some cases of very high heat, can turn them rancid and send free radicals into the air. This is not good. If you choose the electric heat diffuser, make sure you only use the low heat setting for safety.

Oil Burner, Candle, or Electric Lamp (Not recommended)

Candle diffusers are usually made from ceramic, soapstone, heat-tolerant glass, pottery/clay, or other natural stone. There are usually three parts to a candle diffuser: the frame, or bottom chamber, the tea candle beneath, and the bowl or receptacle on top that holds the drops of essential oils. There are also units that are molded as one unit from ceramic, pottery, glass, or natural stone. In each version a lit tealight heats the oil/water causing the essential oil to evaporate into the room. The caution is that a tea light can burn sensitive oils, causing a toxic smoke to leak into the room and/or coagulate as tar on the top receptacle. If you must use one of these devices, be sure you choose a small tea candle because you want a gentle source of heat to release the oil's scent.

In this instance, you waste your valuable oils because the heat from the element or candle destroys the phytochemical essence of the oil. Therefore, anything you burn this way gives you no therapeutic benefit and it is also dangerous. Essential oils are volatile and can catch fire easily. These devices are just not worth the risk.

The bottom line when shopping for diffusers is that you find one that you like, that you will use, and that fits into your lifestyle. Check the ratings and reviews online and the manufacturer's descriptions. When you purchase a diffuser, make sure it is manufactured electrically correct for your country. Get one that has all the bells and whistles you want or need.

Advice and Precautions for Using Diffusers Safely

If diffusing essential oils makes you feel nauseous, light-headed, or bad, stop diffusing immediately and drink plenty of water. This may be a sign your body is going through a detox and you want to cleanse it before you start diffusing again. Begin slowly and work your way up to longer time frames and stronger mixtures.

Make sure you start small when you blend essential oils. If you want to have a couple of different scents, great. But begin with one drop of each essential oil first. See what happens and only increase the amount after you test your tolerance.

Begin your relationship with diffusing slowly. Start with fifteen minutes the first time and gradually work your way up as your tolerance increases.

Clean out your diffuser before each use to avoid buildup, and especially when you change blends or essential oils.

Don't use a lot of oils together as the multiple mixture of essential oils can overwhelm your senses. Limit your mixes and blends to two to three essential oils per session. Timers are also important to have on a diffuser. Some come equipped with a light, a timer, and even LED light color rotations.

Place the diffuser on a high shelf so the oil and air mixture drops down through the air and fills the room from on high. This also keeps the diffuser out of the reach of children and pets.

In terms of safety, I always guard against running diffusers when children are present and when my pets are roaming about. Children are extremely sensitive to diffused essential oils, so make sure they are not exposed to airborne essential oils for more than one to two minutes at a time if they are under the age of twelve.

Essential oils are generally adult entertainment unless used cautiously, and for limited times when children and pets are present. The exception is using essential oils for children when they have colds, coughs, congestion, or are sick with a cold or the flu. You can use diffusers and humidifiers to help break up their congestion, but again, only one to two minutes at a time depending on their age and tolerance. Do a patch test on your kids before using essential oils in diffusers, humidifiers, or as a steam inhalation. And pay attention to the dilution chart.

Diffuser Dilution

Remember, it is important to not use too much of any essential oil because it can overwhelm the space with too much fragrance. That can result in headaches and a waste of your essential oils. Once again, less is more when it comes to diffusing. Here are some guidelines on how to properly dilute your oils in your diffuser. The diffuser size refers to the amount of water that fills the diffuser.

Diffuser Size	Number of Drops
100 ml	3–5
200 ml	6–10
300 ml	9–12
400 ml	12–15
500 ml	15–20

Diffuser Oil Blends According to Purpose

Below are some diffuser blends you can use listed by the result you desire.

Anxiety Relief

1-1 ratio of lavender and rose

Aromatic

1-1 ratio of eucalyptus and rosemary

Celebration
1-2 ratio of lavender and ylang-ylang

Centering
1-1 ratio of geranium and clary sage

Colds
1-2-2 ratio of eucalyptus, tea tree, and orange

Cooling
1-2 ratio of clary sage and peppermint
(Mint essential oils are usually very cooling.)

Coughs
1-1-1-1 ratio of eucalyptus, tea tree, rosemary, and peppermint

Creativity Blast
2 drops of peppermint

Energy Boost
1-2 ratio of peppermint and lemon

Fear Reduction
2-1 ratio of lavender and clary sage

Flu Relief
1-1-1-1 ratio of peppermint, lavender, tea tree, and rosemary

Grief Easement
1-2 ratio of rose and lavender

Insomnia
2-1-1 ratio of lavender, clary sage, and ylang-ylang

Memory Lane
2-1-1 ratio of lemon, lavender, and peppermint

Pain Relief
1-2 ratio of rosemary and geranium

Peace
1-1-2 ratio of lavender, clary sage, and rose

Relaxation
1-1-1 ratio of ylang-ylang, lavender, and geranium

Romance
1-2-1 ratio of ylang-ylang, lavender, and rose

Soul Soothing
1-2-1 ratio of lavender, clary sage, and ylang-ylang

Stress Relief
1-2-1 ratio of geranium, lavender, and clary sage

Therapeutic/Healing
1-2-2 ratio of rose, lavender, and geranium

Weight Reduction
1-2 ratio of peppermint and rosemary

Seasonal Blends for Diffusers

Each season brings with it new and different sensations. You can match your feelings with these appealing blends for each season.

Summer
2 drops lemon
2 drops lavender
1 drop orange

Fall
1 drop tea tree
2 drops lemon
2 drops clary sage

Winter
2 drops frankincense
1 drop rosemary
1 drop eucalyptus

Spring
2 drops ylang-ylang
1 drop lemon
2 drops geranium

In the next chapter, we'll learn how to make some quick and easy products for the face and body.

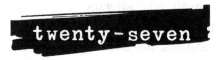

twenty-seven

Application—Basic Recipes for Face and Body

When you begin to use essential oils for the first time, it's a good idea to keep your recipes on the quick and easy side. I've given you a few you can experiment with. Follow them according to the recipe and don't substitute until you know what you are doing. These recipes are successful and satisfying and will keep you exploring more recipes as you enjoy how the products smell and feel on your skin. The best part is that you make them yourself. That's the best reward of all.

Quick Moisturizing Face Cream

To keep your skin feeling fresh, dewy, and supple all day long.

Ingredients

2 oz. of your favorite oil-free lotion

5 drops lavender essential oil

5 drops rosemary essential oil

2 drops sweet orange essential oil*

2 drops Melissa essential oil

2 drops sandalwood essential oil

Directions

Mix together and apply morning and night. Be sure to stir or shake the mixture every time you use it as the essential oils, creams, or lotions can separate. Store in a dark jar out of direct light.

   * Sweet orange is one of the citrus oils that is non-phototoxic if used in this dilution. If you add more than the recommended drops to the cream or lotion, stay out of the sun or sun beds for twelve hours after application.

Quick Wrinkle Cream

There are lots of wrinkle busters in this recipe to help you with aging or maturing skin. It's fast and easy to put together.

Ingredients

2 oz. of your favorite oil-free face cream or lotion

10 drops frankincense essential oil

3 drops rose geranium essential oil

6 drops lavender essential oil

4 drops sandalwood essential oil

3 drops ylang-ylang essential oil

Directions

Mix together and apply morning and night. Be sure to stir or shake the mixture every time you use it as the essential oils, creams, or lotions can separate. Store in a dark jar out of direct light.

Fast Version of a Moisturizing Mask

This mask will give new life to a tired or dry face. Only three ingredients make this quick and easy.

Ingredients

1 Tbsp. sweet almond or jojoba carrier oil
2 drops rose essential oil
2 drops frankincense essential oil

Directions

Mix well and apply to face. Leave on for twenty to thirty minutes and then pat off. Apply Quick Moisturizing Face Cream under makeup or use without makeup.

Oatmeal Bath

For itchy, irritated skin due to rash, eczema, hives, chicken pox, shingles, poison oak, or poison ivy.

Ingredients

1 cup baking soda
1 cup oats
½ cup powdered milk
12 drops lavender essential oil
12 drops Roman chamomile essential oil

6 drops clary sage or frankincense essential oil
Dispersant (Solubol or Polysorbate 20 or 80)

Directions

Combine baking soda, oats, and powdered milk and process into a smooth, fine powder in a blender. Drop by drop, carefully add the essential oils to the mix and blend again. Add dispersant and blend one more time. Store the remedy in a glass (mason) jar away from the light.

Fill a bathtub with lukewarm water. Remove ½ cup of your mixture and allow it to flow into the tub under running water. Stir the bath for proper dispersion and hold the mixture under running water to make sure everything is dispersed thoroughly. Get in and enjoy the relief this oatmeal bath brings you. If some mixture settles to the bottom, stir it up in the water again.

Quick Skin Healing Blend

This is a nice emergency repair recipe for damaged skin from sun, wind, or exposure. It works well in both winter and summer.

Ingredients

4 drops tea tree (or rose geranium or peppermint) essential oil
2 drops rosemary essential oil
1 Tbsp. of carrier oil (olive, jojoba, tamanu, or sweet almond)

Directions

Dilute the tea tree, peppermint, or geranium essential oil in a carrier oil that has anti-inflammatory properties. (Olive, sweet almond, jojoba, avocado, grape seed, pure coconut).

Gently massage your affected skin with the mixture to reduce inflammation. Should you find the blend a bit strong, add more carrier oil to further dilute.

Skin Nourishing Balm

This cream is gentle enough for your face but can be used all over your body for extra-rich nourishing and care.

Ingredients

1 oz. of raw, organic shea, cocoa, or mango butter

5 drops frankincense essential oil

3 drops sandalwood essential oil

2 drops Melissa, Roman chamomile, or rose geranium essential oil

Directions

Carefully heat the shea butter in water using a double boiler—not directly on the stove or over a flame. Remove the pot from the heat, cool slightly, and stir in essential oils. While the mixture is still liquid, pour into a dark glass jar. Allow the mixture to harden at room temperature. Apply the cooled mixture to the undernourished skin.

Summer Sun Cooling Gel

Follow a hot day in the sun with this cooling marvel.

Ingredients

2 oz. aloe vera gel

6 drops lavender essential oil

2 drops rose geranium essential oil

Directions

Mix all the ingredients thoroughly. Transfer the gel into an appropriate container, preferably a glass jar. Store the gel in the refrigerator for better cooling effects. Apply the gel on your skin for cooling and to lessen its itchiness and swelling.

Winter Warming Muscle Balm

Use on those days when your body is cold, tired, and achy after skiing or shoveling snow.

Supplies

Small pot for boiling
Double boiler or pot
Pyrex cup
Funnel
Dark glass container for storage

Ingredients

¼ cup olive, jojoba, sweet almond, or grape seed carrier oil
1 ½ Tbsp. beeswax
8 drops each of the following essential oils:
Peppermint, eucalyptus, clove, thyme, lavender, and Roman chamomile (pre-blend these in a glass cup and set aside)

Directions

Fill your small pot with three to four inches of water and bring to a boil. Carefully insert your double boiler unit or Pyrex cup into the water. Add the carrier oil and beeswax. Stir as the mixture melts. When melted, remove from stove and water, cool for a few moments, and add the essential oils to the mixture.

Stir. Pour the mixture into a dark glass container and allow to cool. The mixture will harden into a nice rub.

At this point, do not wash your instruments. Allow the mixture to harden. If it is too hard for your preference, place it back into the double boiler, gently re-melt the mixture, and add more carrier oil to soften. Be careful not to overheat the essential oils. If it is too runny for you, add another ½ tablespoon of beeswax.

The fragrance of this balm will be much less than that of its retail counterparts. Store in a cool, dark place away from heat and light. Apply as needed for warmth and relief of tired muscles.

Three-Step Easy Calming Salve

This salve calms bites, stings, abrasions, scratches, rug burns, or any minor calamity that is irritated or inflamed.

Ingredients

½ cup jojoba, apricot kernel, or pure coconut oil
1 Tbsp. beeswax
15 drops each lavender and Roman chamomile essential oil

Directions

Melt beeswax and carrier oil in a double boiler. Cool slightly. Add essential oils. Stir and allow to harden in a dark glass jar. If you want a thicker salve, add ½ tablespoon of beeswax to the mix.

All-In-One Cream

This is a cream that's good for just about everything: burns, scratches, dry skin, eczema, you name it. It makes a great morning and night face cream as well as a handy first-aid remedy.

Ingredients

1 Tbsp. apricot kernel oil

1 Tbsp. wheat germ oil

2 tsp. jojoba oil

1 tsp. tamanu or macadamia nut oil

1 tsp. borage oil

½ tsp. carrot seed oil

½ tsp. vitamin E oil

10 drops lavender essential oil

8 drops rose geranium essential oil

8 drops sandalwood essential oil

3 drops rose essential oil

3 drops clary sage essential oil

2 drops ylang-ylang essential oil

2 drops patchouli essential oil

2 drops pine essential oil

2 drops Melissa essential oil

2–4 drops of *your* favorite essential oil, chosen for aroma

½ tsp. vodka or vanilla extract with alcohol

1 Tbsp. pure coconut oil

¼ cup cacao butter

3 Tbsp. shea butter

1 Tbsp. beeswax

¼ cup aloe vera gel

⅔ cup rose hydrosol

Before You Begin

You need to purchase dark glass face cream jars that must be pre-sterilized and cooled. Sterilize your blender with boiling, hot water and allow to dry. Make labels for your jars ahead of time.

Use a double boiler or devise a way to melt ingredients over a hot water bath, like stacking two pots with water in the bottom pot.

Directions

1. Sterilize your containers with hot, boiling water and have them ready and dry.

2. Combine the essential oils, vitamin E, and vodka or vanilla in a small glass container and set aside.

3. Melt cacao butter, shea butter, beeswax, and coconut oil in a double boiler or pan over hot water in a saucepan. Stir together.

4. Allow the mixture to cool a bit, then put in a sterilized blender and add almond, wheat germ, and jojoba oils. Blend on low.

5. Stream in hydrosol and aloe vera gel while on low blend. Blend for a few minutes until mixture thickens.

6. Pour in the essential oil mixture and blend very well (about two to three minutes) until all are completely mixed in.

7. Pour into dry jars and allow mixture to cool before putting on the lids. Add labels.

8. Store extra jars in the refrigerator until use. The first time I made this blend, it had a grainy feeling. When

the mixture sits in your hand, your body heat will soften it. The second time I made it, I blended it for a longer time, and it came out smooth and not grainy. Men and women can use this All-In-One Cream at night or in the morning.

Emergency Dry Skin Face Cream

This cream can be used for those times when your face has been outside and in the elements for a long time.

Ingredients

Use 50 ml or 1.75 oz. of prepared base cream or lotion

2 drops ylang-ylang essential oil

3 drops rose geranium essential oil

3 drops clary sage essential oil

2 drops lavender essential oil

3 drops orange essential oil

Directions

Blend all the ingredients together. Place into a dark glass bottle and store in a cool, dry place.

Essential Oils Moisturizing Mask

When you have a little more time, try this nourishing and moisturizing mask that will leave your face bright, supple, and looking rested.

Ingredients

1 oz. olive, avocado, pomegranate, argan, or sweet almond carrier oil

5 drops rose geranium essential oil
5 drops lavender essential oil
2 drops frankincense essential oil
1 drop clary sage essential oil
2 drops sandalwood essential oil
1 drop patchouli essential oil

Directions

Mix together and store in a dark glass bottle with a stopper or dropper. Shake well before each use. Pour a small dime-size dollop into your hand and massage over your entire face. Leave on for twenty to thirty minutes. (This is a good time to meditate or relax with soft music.) Then wash off. Gently pat dry your face before applying a daytime face cream.

Day Wear for Face

This is a good everyday face prep for under makeup. It keeps your face moisturized and supple all day long.

Ingredients

⅞ oz. apricot kernel oil or carrot seed oil
1 drop frankincense essential oil
1 drop sandalwood essential oil
1 drop lavender essential oil
1 drop Melissa essential oil

Directions

Mix everything together in a one-ounce, dark glass bottle with lid or stopper. Shake vigorously to mix the oils together. (Be sure to shake well before each use.) From the bottle, drop a few drops into the palms of your hands and gently apply to your face. Allow oils to soak in for five minutes before applying makeup.

Night Cream for Face

This provides your skin with wonderful moisturizers that can soak into pores all night for a vibrant look in the morning.

Ingredients

⅞ oz. apricot kernel oil, pomegranate, or carrot seed oil
1 drop frankincense essential oil
2 drops lavender essential oil
1 drop Melissa essential oil
1 drop lemon essential oil
1 drop sandalwood essential oil

Directions

Mix in a one-ounce, dark glass bottle with a dropper/stopper. Shake several times to mix well (shake before each use). Drop a few drops into your palm and rub onto your face. Allow it to soak in for five minutes before going to bed so the oils don't rub off onto bed linens.

There are a lot of recipes for products on the internet. Make sure you read and understand the recipe before you jump in. Some ingredients are hard to find, and others must be ordered from a specialty company. Stick to the basic ingredients for your first few months. When you have mastered these recipes, go ahead and explore. I know I wasted a lot of oils and ingredients in my beginning attempts and I now operate on the side of cautious enthusiasm for all my home-made beauty products.

Making your own creams and salves is a rewarding experience. I wish you well and suggest that a small investment in the proper tools can make all the difference in your level of home success. Most of all, have a good time. You could become the next Elizabeth Arden.

twenty-eight

Using Essential Oils for Body Conditions

W hen we have a physical complaint, many of us go on *automatic* and reach for the medicine cabinet. Now that you have read about the healing properties of essential oils, it may be time to try out a few for your common complaints. Minor injuries, seasonal illnesses, and scrapes and bruises can be helped by using essential oils. Be sure to follow the dilution chart for essential oils and follow the cautions listed for each essential oil in earlier chapters.

With your newly acquired knowledge of essential oils and their benefits, you are probably dying to know how to put them to personal use. In this section we'll explore the various methods of using essential oils and we'll see how essential oils can tackle physical problems in an A–Z format. These are the go-to products I use for maintaining my health and easing discomfort during an illness. I am not suggesting that essential oils replace medical treatment. I believe that they are wonderful preventatives and can work harmoniously alongside traditional medical treatment.

Preventing Illness

It would be safe to say that a good deal of my passion for essential oils comes from the fact that I've been healthy for a very long time. Not becoming susceptible to airborne germs or picking up germs from common handles, doorknobs, and public places is a victory for me. In the past I had a history of tonsillitis (young years) and strep throat, even as an adult. It's been twenty-five years since my last strep throat. I attribute this absence of my previously annual strep to the preventative use of essential oils.

When flying, I carry an inhaler of lavender, eucalyptus, and tea tree essential oils. I use the inhaler several times before, during, and after a flight. I also carry a small vial of homemade hand sanitizer. In the bottle are lavender and lemon essential oils mixed with aloe vera gel. I also carry two small separate vials of lemon and lavender essential oils mixed with antibacterial carrot seed carrier oil. I bring out those vials during the flight, use a few drops, rub into my palms, and inhale. This keeps my sinus passages germ free so I am not affected by the communal air we breathe during a flight. If I am seated next to a germy toddler or someone with a cold, I double my use. I also keep a protective mask in my pocket just in case.

Picking up my luggage, I wipe the handles with my hand sanitizer; and after checking into the hotel, I take out my portable, battery-operated diffuser and cleanse the room with my seasonal mix. I also make sure anything I touch is really clean. It only takes a few minutes to wipe down the phone, remote, doorknobs, handles, and lamp switches. You never know whether the last guest checked out with the flu or pneumonia and left his or her germs all over the devices. Any housekeeper can miss germs left behind on articles in the room. These simple precautions have saved me a lot of down time by preventing a cold, flu, and seasonal illnesses.

You can also carry your purse or pocket kit with you and fight off those germy little invaders before they can even reach you. Refer back to the chapter on blends to find how you can make an inhaler, rollerball, or hand sanitizer. Here I'll also show you how you can make compresses for preventing illnesses and managing them if they arrive.

Compress

Compresses are wonderful aids in healing because essential oils are absorbed by the skin and received by the internal systems of the body via the warmth and water of the compress. If you have a sore throat, upset stomach, strained back, pinched sciatica, bum knee, or chest congestion, you can use a compress to help alleviate the pain and tightness. Essential oils work best with warm compresses, but they can be effective as cold compresses, too.

Medical professionals advise that applied heat brings blood and oxygen to the injured area. The heat can reduce stiffness and muscles spasms when muscles are constricted.

It's not wise to use a heat compress for forty-eight hours following an injury.

Cold Compress: Cold compresses are good for sprains, strains, swelling, pain, and to cool a fever. You can use a compress with ice or just very cold, icy water. Injuries respond best when treated with a cold compress within twenty-four hours of the injury, sprain, or strain. A cold compress numbs the injury, reduces the inflammation, and by lessening the swelling associated with inflammation, reduces the pain of the injury.

You will need

- A small basin
- A tea towel or washcloth
- Some ice and cold water
- Essential oils
- Carrier oil

Directions

1. Fill the basin with two to four cups of cold water.
2. Add ice to cool the water.
3. Once it's gotten very cold, submerge your washcloth or tea towel in the water. Let it chill.
4. While the fabric is cooling, mix anti-inflammatory essential oils with a carrier oil in a proper dilution.
5. Apply that mixture to the area of injury, pain, inflammation, or concern.
6. Wring out the cold towel or washcloth and apply it to the area you are treating.

7. It is recommended you only hold a cold compress on the area for twenty minutes.

Alternatively, you can use crushed ice in a one-quart plastic food storage bag, cover it with a towel, and apply it to the area. A package of frozen peas or corn applied on the area works well, too. You can also dip a tea towel or washcloth in water, place it in a plastic bag, and freeze for fifteen to twenty minutes. When frozen, cover it with another tea towel and apply to the area. Make sure you apply the essential oil mixture to the area you want to treat before applying the cold compress. You can alternate twenty minutes on and twenty minutes off for three rounds to help reduce swelling and discomfort. Wait a few hours before you repeat the process.

Warm Compress #1: There are several ways you can make this compress.

You will need
- A small basin
- A tea towel or washcloth
- Hot or not quite boiling water
- Essential oils
- Carrier oil

Directions
1. Fill the basin with the warm water.
2. Soak the tea towel or washcloth.
3. While it soaks and heats, mix your chosen essential oils with a carrier oil and apply to the spot or area you want to treat. (Follow the dilution chart.)

4. Wring out the towel or washcloth carefully so you don't burn your hands. (When using hot water, be sure it's a safe temperature before applying to the skin. Keep hot water away from small children and pets.)

5. Apply the warm towel to the area you have covered in essential oils and allow it to remain until the towel or washcloth has cooled.

You can repeat this process up to three times and then take a two-hour break to allow the process to work. After the two-hour break, you can repeat the process.

Warm Compress #2: You can add a healing and pain-reducing substance like Epsom salt to the warm water. Use one quarter cup per one cup of water. When it dissolves in the water, soak your towel or washcloth in the mix, wring it out, and apply to the desired area. This is the easiest and most basic compress you can create. Prepare your sore area with diluted essential oils and you can double the healing effect.

If you want to mix essential oils into the hot water, you can, but please use the correct dispersant to make sure the essential oils do not glomp together to avoid a concentrated essential oil accidently getting applied to your skin.

You might also want to use hydrosols in the warmed water. Chamomile hydrosol and calendula hydrosol work to heal broken skin. Bruises and bumps enjoy helichrysum, lavender, and chamomile hydrosols. Sore, strained, and aching muscles respond well to rosemary, eucalyptus, peppermint, and lavender hydrosols.

As with any essential oil product, make sure it is safe for the person using the compress.

Steam Inhalation

The most effective way to get the benefits of an essential oil is to steam inhale it. A steam inhalation is one of the best home remedies for colds and coughs, and it's an effective sinus infection home remedy. Steam inhalations can also be used to relieve sore throats and catarrh.

Steam inhalation is the act of combining essential oils with hot water to create therapeutic steam. Some of the most useful oils for steam inhalation results include eucalyptus, lemon, lavender, rosemary, peppermint, and tea tree.

You will need

- A large pot or heatproof bowl
- 1–2 quarts of boiling water from a kettle or pan
- A large bath towel to cover your head
- Eye protection (closing your eyes super tight will work just as well)
- Essential oils (3–4 drops)
- Dispersant

Directions

1. Heat the water up to boiling on a stove or in an electric kettle.

2. Remove from heat and transfer the water into a large bowl.

3. Add three to four drops of essential oil and dispersant.

4. Cover your head and the bowl with a large bath towel. Position your face above the bowl, but not so close that the steam will burn your face.

5. Inhale the hot steam for several minutes. I do up to five minutes or until the water cools down.

Take caution that you don't burn yourself in this process. Keep children and pets away from the steaming bowl. If you have a cold, a nagging cough, or a chest or sinus infection, steam inhalations can be done several times a day for relief.

A–Z Common Ailments

The following list is a compilation of some of the most common ailments. You can look them up alphabetically and try your hand at healing with nature's beautiful gifts: essential oils. If your illness or injury is serious, you may need medical attention. These suggestions are not intended to replace medical treatment or advice, but as complimentary suggestions for good health. If your symptoms persist or worsen, do seek medical attention.

Acne

Oils beneficial for acne include tea tree, lavender, clary sage, peppermint, and frankincense.

Method 1
Dot any of the above oils on your skin, diluted 1-1.

Method 2

Mix one tablespoon honey, one tablespoon plain yogurt, one tablespoon facial clay mask, and six drops of any of the above oils or a combination of them. Combine all ingredients. Cleanse your face and apply the mixture. Wait one hour before washing off. Repeat every day for three days until inflammation recedes.

Addiction Support

Oils beneficial for addiction support include peppermint, grapefruit, lavender, Roman chamomile, sandalwood, and tangerine.

Method

Use a pendant or a diffuser such as an inhaler that you can access every two hours. Inhale the fragrances singly or combined. Diluted in a massage oil, it can be used for bodily application. Seek additional help with a twelve-step program or physician.

Aging Skin

Oils beneficial for aging skin include lavender, frankincense, sandalwood, ylang-ylang, rose, helichrysum, and geranium.

Method

Mix one ounce of carrier oil (argan, wheat germ, pomegranate, rose hip, neem, borage, macadamia nut, or jojoba) with fifteen drops of frankincense oil and fifteen drops of another essential oil, or a mixture of the oils of your choice from the list above. Mix well and apply to your face, throat, neck, and chest. Use once a day at bedtime for younger-looking and younger-feeling skin.

Allergies

Oils beneficial for allergies include patchouli, Roman chamomile, lavender, peppermint, mandarin orange, eucalyptus, and lemon.

Method

Diffuse three to four drops of a mixture from the above list of essential oils. Or make an inhaler from the list and use every hour for relief.

Anxiety

Oils beneficial for anxiety include lavender, frankincense, Roman chamomile, clary sage, patchouli, geranium, rose, and ylang-ylang.

Method

Use diluted in a massage oil or use a diluted mixture of the above list in an inhaler or diffuser. If you have acute or chronic symptoms of anxiety, always consult a physician.

Arthritis

Oils beneficial for arthritis include eucalyptus, frankincense, lavender, orange, peppermint, rosemary, and thyme.

Method

The best help for arthritis is to reduce the inflammation by creating a rub. Eucalyptus, rosemary, peppermint, and thyme are strong, so be careful you use a proper dilution, especially for use on aging skin. Check the dilution chart and create a rub using a carrier oil (emu, olive, borage, flaxseed) and the correct dilution of any oils from the above list. Try different mixtures until you find the one that provides the most relief for you. Massage the diluted oils onto the sore joints and use a warm compress to enhance the therapeutic value.

Asthma

Oils beneficial for asthma include lavender, peppermint, geranium, clove, eucalyptus, and rosemary. Lavender essential oil is the leading oil recommended during an asthma attack. The rest can be used before and after.

Method 1
Steam inhalation, an inhaler, or a diffuser are your best approaches for asthma relief.

Method 2
Use lavender during an asthma attack in steam inhalation.

Method 3
Use lavender plus geranium, adding clove, eucalyptus, or rosemary in a mix for an inhaler. Use even amounts of drops blended and diluted.

Method 4
Mix two ounces of a carrier oil (flaxseed, grape seed, jojoba, or pomegranate oils) with ten drops of lavender, six drops of geranium, four drops of peppermint, one drop of clove, and

one drop of rosemary. Combine in a dark glass jar. Rub onto chest for relief.

Athlete's Foot

Oils beneficial for athlete's foot include tea tree, lavender, peppermint, eucalyptus, and lemon.

Method

Mix one half ounce of carrier oil with fifteen drops of tea tree, five drops of lavender, and three drops of eucalyptus or lemon. Keep in a dark bottle and drop two to three drops on affected area until symptoms subside. Keep foot exposed to air as much as possible.

Back Pain

Oils beneficial for back pain include Roman chamomile, lavender, peppermint, rosemary, and thyme.

Method

Blend four drops of each essential oil with one ounce of carrier oil (jojoba, borage, olive) and massage into the area of pain. A warm compress placed on the area after the massage may bring relief. For serious back injuries, chronic pain, or if pain does not respond to essential oil treatment, see a physician.

Bad Breath

Oils beneficial for bad breath include peppermint, lemon, and clove.

Method

You will need to take care when using this mouth rinse. Do not swallow. Combine twenty-five to thirty drops of any of the above essential oils with two cups of water. Use this as a rinse two times a day after brushing. Chronic bad breath (halitosis) might be a symptom of a deeper issue. See a physician.

Bleeding Wound

Oils beneficial for a bleeding wound include helichrysum, frankincense, and lavender.

Method

Make sure your wound is not extensive enough to require stitches. If your wound is small and can be treated at home, drop diluted helichrysum onto the small bleeding wound. When the bleeding stops, drop a diluted lavender 1-1 ratio (diluted in an antibacterial carrier oil like jojoba, grape seed, or flaxseed) on the wound. Use diluted frankincense to help the skin heal after the wound is sealed. Dilute with carrier oils suggested above as they have antibacterial and antimicrobial qualities.

Blister

Oils beneficial for blisters include lavender and tea tree.

Method 1

Do not puncture the blister. Cover gently with a piece of cloth soaked in lavender oil diluted in a jojoba, grape seed, or flaxseed carrier oil. Let it sit for twenty minutes. Use the same mixture on a bandage or plaster you use to cover the blister.

Method 2

For foot blisters, you can prepare a footbath using one quart of cool water and twenty drops of tea tree oil. Use a dispersant. Soak your feet for fifteen minutes three times a day until the foot blister is relieved. If blisters show signs of infection, seek medical care as something else may be afoot.

Bronchitis

Oils beneficial for bronchitis include lavender, eucalyptus radiata, rosemary, thyme, and clove.

Method 1

The best way to tackle bronchitis is with a diffuser or steam inhalation. A pocket inhaler is good for the times in between steams. Bronchitis can be a serious condition, so if your symptoms do not respond to this treatment, see a physician. Diffuse lavender, eucalyptus, clove, and rosemary in a diffuser. Diffuse three times a day for thirty minutes for adults.

Method 2

In steam inhalation, use all five oils (five drops each) in a pot of steaming water. Disperse correctly. Inhale these mists three times a day until symptoms are relieved.

Bruise

Oils beneficial for bruises include lavender, helichrysum, frankincense, rosemary, and geranium.

Method

Mix one drop of each essential oil into one tablespoon of jojoba or grape seed carrier oil and apply to bruises. Repeat twice daily for relief and faster healing.

Bug Bites—Bee Sting

Oils beneficial for bites and stings include tea tree, peppermint, and lavender.

Method

Treating insect bites and stings right away helps prevent scratching and infection. Dilute tea tree, rosemary, or peppermint oil in a ratio 1-1 with jojoba oil. Apply to the bite or sting. Repeat every one to two hours. When the sting has subsided, apply diluted lavender oil to the area for skin healing and recovery. (It is a good idea to remove the stinger if present before treating.)

Burns

Oils beneficial for burns include lavender and helichrysum.

Method

Do not use essential oils on second-, third-, or fourth-degree burns. Seek medical help. Use only on minor burns. Dilute lavender oil in a 1-2 mixture with a carrier oil such as jojoba or grape seed. Apply to the burn. When the burn begins to heal, use diluted helichrysum to prevent scarring. You can also mix diluted lavender and helichrysum for the scar-healing process.

Chapped Lips

Oils beneficial for chapped lips include Roman chamomile, lavender, frankincense, rose, and rose geranium.

Method

Make a rollerball with a carrier oil (jojoba, sweet almond, avocado, carrot seed) and mix with two drops of each of the listed essential oils. Mix and roll on lips.

Cold, Prevention

Oils beneficial for cold prevention include orange, pine, eucalyptus, and lavender.

Method

Diffuse a blend of these essential oils twice daily during cold and flu season.

Cold, Symptoms Relief/Congestion

Oils beneficial for cold symptoms relief and congestion include eucalyptus, lemon, thyme, clove, and rosemary.

Method 1

The best relief of cold symptoms is to use steam inhalation twice a day. You can also create an inhaler and take it with you. Use every hour to relieve symptoms.

Method 2

For the inhaler, use three drops of each oil from the above list in a carrier oil.

Cough

Oils beneficial for coughs include eucalyptus, tea tree, thyme, rosemary, peppermint, and lemon.

Method

Create a steam inhalation blend with the above list. Inhale deeply and use this method three times a day.

Dandruff

Oils beneficial for dandruff include patchouli, tea tree, lavender, thyme, peppermint, Roman chamomile, and rosemary.

Method 1

Add ten drops of any of the essential oils to your shampoo each time you wash your hair. Do not combine with entire shampoo bottle. One serving at a time.

Method 2

Mix forty drops in any combination of the above list in one ounce of carrier oil, (apricot kernel, sweet almond, pure coconut). Massage into scalp. Cover with a shower cap and wait one hour. Wash hair after one hour. Repeat treatment two to three times a week until dandruff is gone. Dandruff is usually caused by yeast or fungus, environment, diet, or hair products.

Depression

Oils beneficial for depression include lavender, ylang-ylang, patchouli, bergamot, Roman chamomile, sandalwood, orange, clary sage, geranium, and rose.

Method

Diffusing any of the oils listed above, blending them, or using them individually is a great way to begin. Start with a blend of three oils and experiment. For a quick lift, blend orange, lavender, and sandalwood.

Note: Each of us is biochemically different. The blend that works for one may not work for another. The way to know what works for you is through trial and error.

Dermatitis

Oils beneficial for dermatitis include peppermint, Roman chamomile, frankincense eucalyptus, lemon, lavender, and tea tree.

Method

Combine the drops of any of the above (see dilution chart) with carrot seed carrier oil and rub into skin two to three times daily until the condition improves.

Dry Skin

Oils beneficial for dry skin include lavender, helichrysum, geranium, frankincense, and sandalwood.

Method

Combine drops of any of the above (see dilution chart) with carrot seed, rose hip, avocado, grape seed, jojoba, pomegranate, safflower, or sweet almond carrier oil and rub into skin two to three times daily until the condition improves.

Ear Infection

Oils beneficial for an ear infection include tea tree, lavender, and thyme.

Method

Blend one drop of each oil listed above with jojoba carrier oil. Saturate a cotton ball with half the mixture and place the cotton ball in the outer ear canal. Do not push into ear. Rub the rest of the diluted mixture around the outside of the ear. Do not do this procedure if ear drum has ruptured. Seek medical help.

Fibromyalgia

Oils beneficial for fibromyalgia include lavender, peppermint, sandalwood, eucalyptus, and clove.

Method 1

Combine three drops of each oil listed above with one ounce of carrier oil (avocado, jojoba, rose hip, olive, borage) and use as a massage tool for relief of pain.

Method 2

Use a blend of three of the oils listed above in a diffuser and inhale two to three times a day.

Fleas

Oils beneficial for flea control include lavender, lemon, peppermint, rosemary, clove, and pine.

Method 1
For prevention and to get rid of fleas, prepare a spray with three drops of each oil listed above in eight ounces of water. Test area for staining first. Remove pets and children from the area. Spray carpet, furniture, rugs, and pet beds. *Do not spray on pets.* Allow area to dry before allowing children or pets access.

Method 2
Combine three drops of each essential oil listed above and add one half ounce carrier oil. Soak cotton balls in the mixture and place in areas where fleas enter. Do not leave where children or pets can access the balls. Use a mesh jewelry bag to keep little hands and paws away from the cotton balls soaked in essential oils.

Flu
Oils beneficial for flu include thyme, eucalyptus, frankincense, peppermint, lemon, tea tree, clove, and rosemary.

Method
Select any of the oils listed above and diffuse in your room to prevent the flu or help heal it if you catch it. Clean surfaces, doorknobs, handles, and counters with lemon oil and water to keep germs at bay. Use any of the essential oils listed above to make an inhaler to reduce symptoms or prevent the flu germs from reaching you. Use a blend of the above oils in a carrier oil for a feel-better massage.

Grief

Oils beneficial for grief include bergamot, lemon, rose, frankincense, geranium, and lavender.

Method

There are many stages of grief ranging from shock, denial, anger, and exhaustion and all the emotions in between. Keep essential oils close by in a diffuser, inhaler, rollerball, warm bath, or cotton balls soaked with the essence. You will experience the gamut of emotions and select the one that works for you at each stage. Eventually the grief will lessen, and you will be ready for joyful orange.

Hair Loss

Oils beneficial for hair loss include ylang-ylang, peppermint, rosemary, clary sage, thyme, tea tree, and lavender.

Method

If you experience hair loss, you can begin to prevent it by increasing scalp health. Add a few drops of any of the above essential oils to your shampoo to keep your scalp and hair healthy. For an intense treatment, add fifteen drops (total) of the above essential oils to one ounce of shampoo and wait one hour before shampooing. Repeat this process three times a week until you notice improvement.

Headache

Oils beneficial for headaches include lavender, peppermint, eucalyptus, frankincense, and rosemary.

Method 1

There are many ways to relieve a headache. Make an inhaler with the above essential oils.

Method 2

Blend them together for a warm compress. Use them mixed with a carrier oil for a massage.

Method 3

Diffuse any blend of the above list.

Method 4

Create a rollerball and roll the diluted mixture onto your temples, wrists, and the back of your neck.

Method 5

Take a warm bath with properly dispersed essential oils. Do all the above until you experience relief.

Heartburn

Oils beneficial for heartburn include eucalyptus and peppermint.

Method

Do not ingest. Make a blend of one or two of these essential oils (six drops) mixed in two teaspoons of carrier oil. Massage on the upper chest and stomach, clockwise.

Hives

Oils beneficial for hives include peppermint, lavender, tea tree, Roman chamomile, helichrysum, and frankincense.

Method

Dilute any of the above essential oils in a 1-2 ratio and dab with a cotton ball onto breakout. If there is any irritation, wipe off with olive oil and try another blend. Peppermint and tea tree are the most likely to cause a reaction, so have the olive oil or a carrier oil standing by. Roman chamomile, lavender, and helichrysum are the mildest. Follow dilution directions for children.

Insect Repellant

Oils beneficial for insect repellant include geranium, eucalyptus, thyme, peppermint, tea tree, clove, and lavender.

Method 1 (General)

Add twenty-four drops total of any of the above or eight drops each of three essential oils. Mix into four ounces of witch hazel (non-alcohol, non-paraben). Pour blend into a spray bottle and shake well. You will need to apply every couple of hours. Spray clothes and skin for best protection. Avoid spraying into eyes.

Method 2 (General)

Another blend: twenty-four drops each of patchouli and geranium essential oils. Mix in a spray bottle with four ounces of water. Shake well and store in a dark place. Apply every couple of hours. Do not allow the mixture to sit in the sun. Avoid spraying into eyes.

Method 3 (Mosquitos)

Oils beneficial for mosquito repellant include citronella, peppermint, lemon, eucalyptus, clove, thyme, geranium, and lavender.

Method 4 (Fleas)
Oils beneficial for flea repellant include citronella, eucalyptus, tea tree, lavender, orange, and pine.

Method 5 (Ticks)
Oils beneficial for tick repellant include geranium and thyme. Never spray any of these repellants on pets or children under twelve.

Insomnia
Oils beneficial for insomnia include lavender, ylang-ylang, Roman chamomile, clary sage, sandalwood, and bergamot.

Method 1
Any of the above essential oils are relaxing and can help you achieve a state of rest. You can use one or a combination in a warm bath, properly dispersed.

Method 2
You can use a warm compress on your head and back of neck using this list. You can diffuse up to three of these essential oils just before bed to relax you and bring on sleep.

Method 3
You can also make an inhaler with a combination of the above and use that to bring on relaxation and induce sleep.

Joint Pain
Oils beneficial for joint pain include peppermint, eucalyptus, rosemary, clove, thyme, frankincense, and lavender.

Method

All the above oils (except lavender and frankincense) tend to be "hot" oils and they need proper dilution. Test your mixture before applying to your skin. Combine a hot oil with a cooler oil and dilute in a carrier oil (emu, olive, borage, flaxseed, jojoba) for an even blend.

Cover your joint with this rub and apply a warm compress. With or without the compress, these mixes are meant to bring you comfort and relief from inflammation. See recipe section for additional rubs and pain relievers.

Knee Pain

See above.

Leg Cramps

Oils beneficial for leg cramps include peppermint, lavender, thyme, eucalyptus, clary sage, and Roman chamomile.

Method

Use a rub, soak in a bath, or use a compress to relieve leg cramps. Mix ten drops of an essential oil (or combination of the above) in one ounce of carrier oil and use as a rub, in a bath properly dispersed, or in a warm compress.

Lice

Oils beneficial for lice include tea tree, lavender, neem, clove, eucalyptus, and thyme.

Method

Mix fifteen to twenty drops of essential oil into two ounces of olive oil or almond oil. Massage onto head or scalp. Leave on hair for twelve hours. Comb one section at a time to remove lice and eggs from head. Shampoo hair. Refrain from using a conditioner until you are sure all lice are gone. You can repeat this process up to three times, if needed.

Low Testosterone Support

Oils beneficial for low testosterone include ylang-ylang, clary sage, and peppermint.

Method 1

Diffuse during the day.

Method 2

Create a warm bath using any or all the essential oils listed above, dispersed correctly.

Make a massage blend in correct dilution and massage the body, especially the chest, abdomen, back, and legs. Do not use on genitals.

Menopause

Oils beneficial for menopause include clary sage, geranium, lavender, peppermint, and citrus.

Method 1

Combine any of the above oils and properly disperse in a warm, relaxing bath.

Method 2

Use as a diluted blend in a cool compress for hot flashes.

Method 3

Use in a diffuser to help relax and relieve discomfort.

Migraine

Oils beneficial for migraines include lemon, lavender, rosemary, eucalyptus, and geranium.

Method

Use in a diffuser, steam inhaler, warm bath, cool or hot compress, inhaler, or rollerball for massage oil. Use these essential oils in blends of three, diluted with a carrier oil for all the above. Do not use a carrier oil in the diffuser.

Morning Sickness

Oils beneficial for morning sickness include peppermint, lavender, and lemon. (Do not use in first trimester.)

Method

Use in a diffuser, steam inhaler, warm bath, cool or hot compress, inhaler, or rollerball for massage oil. Use these essential oils in a blend. Dilute accordingly.

Muscle Aches

Oils beneficial for muscle aches include peppermint, eucalyptus, rosemary, lavender, helichrysum, clove, thyme, frankincense, and pine.

Method 1
Use thyme in a warm carrier oil. Rub onto sore muscles. Mix pine and lavender in a carrier oil (jojoba or sweet almond) and rub into achy muscles.

Method 2
Create a warm compress of peppermint, eucalyptus, and lavender and alternate with ice pack: twenty minutes on, twenty minutes off. Repeat three times and rest.

Nail Care
Oil beneficial for nail care includes lavender.

Method
Mix wheat germ oil with lavender and massage into nails and fingertips.

Nail Fungus
Oils beneficial for nail fungus include tea tree, clove, and patchouli.

Method
Mix two drops of tea tree oil, two drops of clove, and one drop of patchouli. Add to one teaspoon of carrier oil. Drop onto affected toes and nails. Allow oil to penetrate. Keep affected toes and nails open to the air as much as possible. Repeat three times a day until symptoms subside.

Nausea
Oils beneficial for nausea include lavender and peppermint.

Method

Create a rollerball with a mix of both oils and a carrier oil. Roll onto abdomen and under nose. Create a blend of the essential oils and use as a cold compress on the abdomen or neck and chest until symptoms subside. If nausea is accompanied by vomiting, you may need to see a medical professional.

Neck Pain

Oils beneficial for neck pain include peppermint, eucalyptus, rosemary, lavender, helichrysum, clove, thyme, frankincense, and pine.

Method 1

Use thyme in a warm carrier oil. Rub onto sore neck muscles.

Method 2

Mix pine and lavender in a carrier oil (jojoba and sweet almond) and rub onto back of neck muscles.

Method 3

Create a warm compress of peppermint, eucalyptus, and lavender.

Nervousness

Oils beneficial for nervousness include clary sage, lavender, bergamot, Roman chamomile, and rose.

Method 1

Make an inhaler blending the above list. Use in a diffuser, or in a massage blend.

Method 2
Use in a warm bath properly dispersed.

Method 3
A roller blend is great for rolling on temples, wrists, and back of neck. Seek medical care if nervous condition persists.

Oily Skin
Oils beneficial for oily skin include lavender and lemon.

Method
Mix seven drops of lemon and five drops of lavender with one ounce of vodka or witch hazel. Massage mixture onto clean skin. If 190-proof vodka is too drying for your skin, use witch hazel instead. Repeat two times a day until you see results. Not for use on children.

Pneumonia
Oils beneficial for pneumonia include lavender, eucalyptus, thyme, tea tree, peppermint, and clove.

Method 1
Use in steam inhalation, an inhaler, or a warm bath with properly dispersed essential oils to help symptoms. A warm chest compress and a diffuser also helps.

Method 2
Use a blend of the above and use a carrier oil to dilute. If symptoms persist, seek medical care. Pneumonia is a serious condition.

Premenstrual Syndrome (PMS)

Oils beneficial for PMS include clary sage, lavender, geranium, and rose.

Method

Add ten drops of clary sage to proper dispersant and enjoy a warm bath. You can mix lavender, geranium, and rose with a proper dispersant and do the same thing. A warm compress helps on the lower abdomen using the same essential oils.

Poison Ivy

Oils beneficial for poison ivy include lavender, tea tree, eucalyptus, peppermint, frankincense, helichrysum, and Roman chamomile.

Method 1

Make an oatmeal bath using a combination of the above oils. (See recipes under Oatmeal Bath.)

Method 2

Blend eight drops of helichrysum and four drops of lavender with two ounces of aloe vera gel. Gently apply to the affected skin area.

Psoriasis

Oils beneficial for psoriasis include lavender, helichrysum, Roman chamomile, bergamot, sandalwood, patchouli, and germanium.

Method 1
Use a combination of fifty drops of essential oils in one half cup of carrier oil (argan or pure coconut). Mix well and apply to affected skin.

Method 2
Use in a compress, as a rub, or in a massage to calm the itchy, red sores. Repeat application three times a day until symptoms subside.

Restless Leg Syndrome (RLS)
Oils beneficial for RLS include lavender, Roman chamomile, and frankincense.

Method 1
Diffuse a blend of the above oils.

Method 2
Bathe in a warm bath with properly dispersed essential oils from the list above. Create warm compresses and wrap your legs in frankincense and jojoba oil.

Ringworm
Oils beneficial for ringworm include geranium, eucalyptus, peppermint, thyme, lavender, and tea tree.

Method
Mix equal amounts of any three essential oils and an equal amount of a carrier oil (pomegranate, pure coconut, sweet almond, or jojoba) in a 1-1-1 ratio. Apply to the affected area

with a cotton ball or swab. Dispose of the cotton ball immediately. Repeat two times a day until the ringworm fades. Do not use on pets.

Scalp Psoriasis

Oils beneficial for scalp psoriasis include carrot seed, lavender, and tea tree.

Method

Combine ten drops of a combination of the essential oils with one tablespoon of carrier oil (carrot seed or argan) and massage mixture on damp, clean hair onto the scalp. Wait thirty minutes and then shampoo. Repeat this process three times a day until symptoms disappear.

Scabies

Oils beneficial for scabies include clove, tea tree, and peppermint.

Method

Mix twenty drops of any of the above essential oils with aloe vera or neem carrier oil. Apply the blend to the affected area. Repeat treatment two times a day for three days. Repeat as needed until parasites are gone. You will also need to wash linens, bedding, and clothing with ten drops of tea tree oil added to wash.

Scarring

Oils beneficial for scars include helichrysum, lavender, frankincense, and geranium.

Method

Mix twenty-four drops of any one or a combination of the above essential oils with two tablespoons of carrot seed or rose hip carrier oil. Apply morning and night to scarred area.

Seasonal Affective Disorder (SAD)

Oils beneficial for SAD include orange, peppermint, and bergamot.

Method

Diffuse a blend of six drops of each oil listed above to lift your mood.

Shingles

Oils beneficial for shingles include peppermint, geranium, thyme, lemon, and clove.

Method

Add a combination of eight drops of essential oil to one teaspoon carrier oil (pure coconut, sweet almond, or argan). Test on inflamed skin. If it's too harsh or it stings, add more carrier oil. Repeat treatment four to five times a day until symptoms subside. If you have a severe case, seek medical attention.

Sinusitis

Oils beneficial for sinusitis include peppermint, rosemary, eucalyptus, thyme, and lemon.

Method 1

Steam inhale a blend of five oils dispersed in hot water. Inhale for five minutes.

Method 2

Diffuse all five essential oils for twenty minutes, three times a day.

Method 3

Create an inhaler of the blend and use once an hour.

Smoking Cessation

Oils beneficial for smoking cessation include lavender, Roman chamomile, ylang-ylang, lemon, and orange.

Method 1

Use essential oils from the above list in an inhaler or in a diffuser to help quell the cravings.

Method 2

Use lavender, Roman chamomile, and ylang-ylang to calm your nerves in an inhaler blend or in a diffuser.

Method 3

Use orange or lemon, or both, to lift and brighten your mood in an inhaler or in a diffuser.

Sore Throat

Oils beneficial for sore throat include eucalyptus, tea tree, peppermint, thyme, and lemon.

Method

Sore throats are best treated with a diffuser or steam inhalation. Use a combination of the above essential oils in a blend or use them individually to ease and heal a sore throat. If your sore throat continues, you may need to seek medical help.

Sprain

Oils beneficial for sprains include frankincense, peppermint, pine, and eucalyptus.

Method 1

For minor sprains, use any of the above essential oils in a cold compress for relief. Apply three times a day until swelling subsides.

Method 2

Make a special salve using eight drops of any or all of the above essential oils in one teaspoon carrier oil (flaxseed, grape seed, or jojoba) and apply to injured area. Elevate limb. If there is discoloration or a broken bone, seek medical attention.

Stiff Neck

Oils beneficial for neck stiffness include clary sage, rosemary, and lavender.

Method

Dilute all three in a carrier oil and apply to neck. Use a warm compress for relief.

Stress Management

Oils beneficial for stress management include lavender, clary sage, bergamot, Roman chamomile, ylang-ylang, and rose.

Method

Diffusers are great for reducing stress. Choose any of the above or a blend and diffuse several times a day. Inhalers using a blend of the above can be handy for a quick stress breaker. The above list of oils can help release tightness when mixed in carrier oils for a massage.

Stretch Marks

Oils beneficial for stretch marks include helichrysum, frankincense, lavender, and geranium.

Method

Mix twenty-four drops of any one or a combination of the above essential oils with two tablespoons of carrot or grape seed or rose hip carrier oil. Apply morning and night to stretch mark area.

Sunburn

Oils beneficial for sunburn include peppermint, geranium, eucalyptus, tea tree, lavender, Roman chamomile, vitamin E, and vitamin C.

Method

Mix ten drops of peppermint oil in ten ounces of water, add to a sprayer, shake well, and spray on the burned area. (You can use tea tree or eucalyptus in place of peppermint.) Once the burn has cooled from the peppermint, you can make another spray bottle of water and lavender and Roman chamomile: five drops of each oil to ten ounces of water. Spray again with this mixture.

Swelling

Oils beneficial for swelling include eucalyptus, lavender, peppermint, Roman chamomile, and rosemary.

Method

Mix one tablespoon of carrier oil with twenty drops of the above selection. Massage onto the swollen area. Use a cold compress on top of the rub for relief. If there is dark discoloration or you suspect a broken bone, seek medical attention.

Tendinitis

Oils beneficial for tendinitis include eucalyptus and peppermint.

Method

Blend four drops of each essential oil with one teaspoon of carrier oil (avocado, sweet almond, or olive). Apply to inflamed tendon area. Apply a cold compress to area, elevate, and rest. Repeat three times a day. If pain or swelling increases, seek medical attention.

Toothache

Oils beneficial for toothaches include lemon, clove, and Roman chamomile.

Method 1

Clove essential oil can numb the pain while you await your dental appointment. Use only one drop. Apply to tooth with a toothpick. Do not swallow. Wait two minutes. Wipe off remainder so you do not ingest. You can repeat this process three times a day.

Method 2

To reduce jaw ache, blend two drops of each of the above listed oils in one teaspoon carrier oil and massage onto painful area of the jaw.

Varicose Veins

Oils beneficial for varicose veins include lavender, rosemary, helichrysum, frankincense, lemon, and geranium.

Method 1

Blend four drops of lavender and rosemary with one teaspoon of carrier oil and massage onto bulging veins.

Method 2

Blend two drops each of helichrysum, frankincense, lemon, and geranium in one teaspoon of carrier oil and massage onto area.

Weight-Loss Support

Oil beneficial for weight-loss support includes clove.

Method

Create an inhaler with close essential oil and use twenty minutes before mealtime. Diffuse this blend twenty minutes before mealtime to curb the appetite.

Wrinkles

Oils beneficial for wrinkles include helichrysum, lavender, geranium, and frankincense.

Method

Mix five drops of each listed oil in one ounce of carrier oil (rose hip, neem, apricot kernel, pomegranate, borage, macadamia nut, or tamanu) or face lotion and apply to clean skin at bedtime. Cover face, neck, and chest area for best results.

Yeast Infection

Oils beneficial for yeast infection include tea tree, thyme, geranium, lavender, clove, and patchouli.

Note: There is an exception here to using essential oils on genitalia as they are well-diluted in yogurt. Follow the recipe exactly.

Method 1 (Women)

Mix two drops each of lavender, tea tree, and patchouli in four ounces of yogurt. Apply to interior of vagina once a day.

Method 2 (Men)

Mix two drops each of tea tree and patchouli in two tablespoons of carrier oil (grape seed, jojoba, or pure coconut) and massage on penis under foreskin two times a day.

The uses for essential oils have been handed down for centuries through many civilizations and a panoply of healers. Some remedies may work wonderfully for you, while others may seem ineffective. You alone will be the judge. The importance of using pure and organic essential and carrier oils should be more than obvious to you after reading the above remedies. Keep your essential oils and carrier oils up to date, well preserved, and in top form, and you should see how remarkable they can be for assisting with healing and symptom reduction. If you think you need medical attention, seek it right away.

In the next chapter we will venture into the world of emotional uses for our beloved essential oils.

twenty-nine

Using Essential Oils for Mind and Emotions

In the last chapter we explored how we can use essential oils to help us heal our physical complaints and bodily needs. Essential oils are not limited to the physical; they can also help with our mental and emotional states. I can't begin to count the number of times I have come home from a stressful day, or had a disagreement with a friend or colleague, and needed a little help to adjust my emotions back into alignment.

There isn't one of us who doesn't need an occasional shoulder to cry on, a sympathetic ear to hear our woes, or a gentle, reassuring touch. That's what essential oils can do for us when our best friend isn't around. In fact, in many ways they are our best friends.

There were times when I reached for a glass of wine to relax, but I think I am happiest and feel the most healed and content when I relax in the company of my essential oils and their wonderful, transporting aromas.

Based on my personal experience and research, I've put together a list of essential oils that might improve the various emotional states we all experience at one time or another. You can use this as a reference and make your own blends using these suggestions. Or, you can go along with the sample recipe for blends that cover a wide range of emotional scenarios. You'll find everything from grief to celebration in the lists below. I hope you'll try them all when the opportunity presents.

This is a sampling of recipes and ideas to get you started and stir your creative juices. As you test them, some will smell terrific to you and others may not be to your liking. You are invited to create your own. Live your beautiful life on the wings of your personal preference and use these oils in accordance with how they make you *feel*.

A journal or a notebook is a wonderful tool to help you remember what works for you and what doesn't. I recommend you start one right away to record your explorations, like a travel log. You may adore some of the combinations, or you may not like them at all. Remember, there's never a bad blend; only a personal preference. If a scent is too floral for you, then add some of the Base notes you learned about in chapter 25. If it is too heavy, add some Top or Middle notes.

Acceptance and Forgiveness

If you are having difficulty accepting things the way they are, or if you need to forgive someone or something to move on, these essential oils will help you heal and move forward.

Recommended Oils

Bergamot, lavender, lemon, Melissa, rose, ylang-ylang

Sample Recipes for Acceptance and Forgiveness

#1

1 oz. carrier oil

2 drops rose essential oil

1 drop bergamot essential oil

1 drop lemon essential oil

1 drop Melissa essential oil

Use as a massage oil blend.

#2

1 oz. carrier oil

2 drops lemon essential oil

2 drops ylang-ylang essential oil

1 drop rose essential oil

Use as a massage oil blend.

#3

For diffuser:

2 drops Melissa essential oil

2 drops bergamot essential oil

1 drop rose essential oil

1 drop lavender

Anger and Temper

When you are angry or tend to lose your temper, these essential oils can help you cope.

Recommended Oils

Bergamot, orange, patchouli, Roman chamomile, rose, ylang-ylang

Sample Recipes for Anger and Temper

#1

1–2 oz. carrier oil

1 drop rose essential oil

3 drops orange essential oil

1 drop patchouli essential oil

1 drop Roman chamomile essential oil

Use as a massage oil blend. Use any of these combinations in a diffuser, minus the carrier oil, if you prefer inhalation.

#2

1 oz. carrier oil

2 drops Roman chamomile essential oil

2 drops ylang-ylang essential oil

1 drop orange essential oil

1 drop rose essential oil

Use as a massage oil blend.

#3

For diffuser:

3 drops rose essential oil

2 drops ylang-ylang essential oil

2 drops bergamot essential oil

Anxiety and Stress

If you find yourself in a situation that is stressful or you have anxiety about it, this group of essential oils were made to help you manage those emotions.

Recommended Oils

Bergamot, clary sage, frankincense, geranium, lavender, patchouli, rose, sandalwood

Sample Recipes for Anxiety and Stress

#1

1 oz. carrier oil
2 drops bergamot essential oil
2 drops clary sage essential oil
1 drop frankincense essential oil
1 drop geranium essential oil
1 drop rose essential oil
Use as a massage oil blend.

#2

1 oz. carrier oil
1 drop patchouli essential oil
2 drops lavender essential oil
1 drop clary sage essential oil
1 drop sandalwood essential oil
2 drops orange essential oil
Use as a massage oil blend.

#3

For diffuser:
9 drops lavender essential oil
6 drops clary sage essential oil
2 drops sandalwood essential oil

Concentration

If you want to improve your concentration and focus, use the following essential oils to sharpen your mind and bring clarity.

Recommended Oils
Clove, eucalyptus, lemon, peppermint, rosemary, tea tree

Sample Recipe for Concentration
#1
1 oz. carrier oil
1 drop lemon essential oil
3 drops rosemary essential oil
2 drops clove essential oil
1 drop peppermint essential oil
Use as a massage oil blend.

#2
1 oz. carrier oil
2 drops peppermint essential oil
2 drops lemon essential oil
1 drop rosemary essential oil
1 drop tea tree essential oil
Use as a massage oil blend.

#3
For diffuser:
2 drops rosemary essential oil
1 drop clove essential oil
1 drop eucalyptus essential oil
1 drop lemon essential oil

Depression and Despondency

For short-term feelings of being blue or down in the dumps, these essential oils can help lift your spirits and remind you of the good things in life.

Recommended Oils

Bergamot, clary sage, frankincense, geranium, lavender, lemon, Melissa, orange, Roman chamomile, rose, sandalwood, ylang-ylang

Sample Recipe for Depression and Despondency

#1

1 oz. carrier oil
2 drops frankincense essential oil
1 drop lemon essential oil
2 drops ylang-ylang essential oil
1 drop bergamot essential oil
2 drops pine essential oil
Use as a massage oil blend.

#2

1 oz. carrier oil
1 drop geranium essential oil
1 drop rose essential oil
3 drops lavender essential oil
Use as a massage oil blend.

#3

For diffuser:
2 drops lavender essential oil
1 drop frankincense essential oil
1 drop orange essential oil
1 drop sandalwood essential oil
1 drop geranium essential oil

Exhaustion and Mental Fatigue

For those instances when you are burned out and mentally tired, these essential oils can give you the boost you need to carry on.

Recommended Oils
Bergamot, clary sage, eucalyptus, frankincense, lemon, peppermint, pine, rosemary

Sample Recipe for Exhaustion and Mental Fatigue
#1
1 oz. carrier oil
2 drops bergamot essential oil
1 drop eucalyptus essential oil
2 drops lemon essential oil
1 drop peppermint essential oil
Use as a massage oil blend.

#2
1 oz. carrier oil
2 drops peppermint essential oil
1 drop frankincense essential oil
3 drops lemon essential oil
1 drop clary sage essential oil
Use as a massage oil blend.

#3
For diffuser:
2 drops peppermint essential oil
2 drops frankincense essential oil
1 drop bergamot essential oil

Fear

The following essential oils help you relax and quell those fears that freeze you in your tracks. You can overcome almost anything using these oils.

Recommended Oils

Bergamot, clary sage, frankincense, lemon, Roman chamomile, lavender, orange, pine, sandalwood

Sample Recipes for Fear

#1

1 oz. carrier oil
3 drops sandalwood essential oil
2 drops orange essential oil
1 drop clary sage essential oil
1 drop pine essential oil
Use as a massage oil blend.

#2

1 oz. of carrier oil
2 drops clary sage essential oil
2 drop roman chamomile essential oil
1 drop pine essential oil
2 drops lavender essential oil
Use as a massage oil blend.

#3

For diffuser:
2 drops bergamot essential oil
2 drops orange essential oil
1 drop sandalwood essential oil

Irritability

When certain people or things get on your nerves, use these essential oils to alleviate those feelings.

Recommended Oils

Lavender, lemon, sandalwood, patchouli, Roman chamomile, pine

Sample Recipes for Irritability

#1

1 oz. carrier oil
2 drops lavender essential oil
4 drops sandalwood essential oil
2 drops Roman chamomile essential oil
Use as a massage oil blend.

#2

1 oz. of carrier oil
2 drops lavender essential oil
1 drop lemon essential oil
2 drops Roman chamomile essential oil
1 drop patchouli essential oil
Use as a massage oil blend.

#3

For diffuser:
2 drops Roman chamomile essential oil
2 drops sandalwood essential oil
1 drop lavender essential oil
1 drop lemon essential oil

Loss and Grief

Recovering from a loss and dealing with the grief associated with loss is difficult. Things do get better with time and these essential oils.

Recommended Oils

Frankincense, helichrysum, lavender, rose, sandalwood

Sample Recipes for Loss and Grief

#1

1 oz. carrier oil
1 drop frankincense essential oil
1 drop helichrysum essential oil
1 drop lavender essential oil
2 drops sandalwood essential oil
Use as a massage oil blend.

#2

1 oz. carrier oil
2 drops rose essential oil
3 drops sandalwood essential oil
1 drop helichrysum essential oil
Use as a massage oil blend.

#3

For diffuser:
1 drop rose essential oil
2 drops helichrysum essential oil
1 drop frankincense essential oil
1 drop lavender essential oil

Panic Attacks

If life's challenges or situations cause you panic attacks, you can manage those emotions with these essential oils.

Recommended Oils

Lavender, Melissa, Roman chamomile, patchouli, rose, sandalwood

Sample Recipes for Panic Attacks

#1

1 oz. carrier oil

2 drops lavender essential oil

2 drops sandalwood essential oil

1 drop rose essential oil

1 drop Roman chamomile essential oil

Use as a massage oil blend.

#2

1 oz. carrier oil

2 drops lavender essential oil

2 drops Melissa essential oil

1 drop patchouli essential oil

1 drop Roman chamomile essential oil

Use as a massage oil blend.

#3

For diffuser:

2 drops lavender essential oil

2 drops Melissa essential oil

1 drop rose essential oil

Peace and Happiness

Sometimes we can all use a little help from our friends to establish a moment of calm.

Recommended Oils

Bergamot, frankincense, geranium, lemon, Melissa, orange, pine, rose, ylang-ylang

Sample Recipes for Peace and Happiness

#1

1 oz. carrier oil
1 drop Melissa essential oil
2 drops frankincense essential oil
2 drops orange essential oil
1 drop ylang-ylang essential oil
1 drop rose essential oil
Use as a massage oil blend.

#2

1 oz. carrier oil
3 drops bergamot essential oil
2 drops ylang-ylang essential oil
1 drop rose essential oil
1 drop lemon essential oil
Use as a massage oil blend.

#3

For diffuser:
2 drops orange essential oil
1 drop rose essential oil
2 drops Melissa essential oil

Self-Esteem

If you don't feel confident about yourself in a given moment, these essential oils are here to help boost your self-confidence.

Recommended Oils

Bergamot, lavender, lemon, peppermint, rose, orange, spearmint, geranium, frankincense

Sample Recipes for Self-Esteem

#1

1 oz. carrier oil
2 drops lavender essential oil
2 drops bergamot essential oil
1 drop rose essential oil
1 drop frankincense essential oil
Use as a massage oil blend.

#2

1 oz. carrier oil
2 drops lavender essential oil
2 drops geranium essential oil
1 drop frankincense essential oil
1 drop sweet orange essential oil
Use as a massage oil blend.

#3

For diffuser:
2 drops lavender essential oil
2 drops geranium essential oil
1 drop rose essential oil
1 drop lemon essential oil.

Stress

For when you're at the end of your rope and your nerves are frayed, employ these essential oils to help you return to a balanced emotional state.

Recommended Oils

Bergamot, clary sage, rose, geranium, lavender, Melissa, patchouli, Roman chamomile, ylang-ylang

Sample Recipes for Stress

#1

1 oz. carrier oil
3 drops bergamot essential oil
2 drops clary sage essential oil
2 drops Roman chamomile essential oil
1 drop geranium essential oil
Use as a massage oil blend.

#2

1 oz. carrier oil
7 drops ylang-ylang essential oil
4 drops lavender essential oil
5 drops patchouli essential oil
1 drop Melissa essential oil
Use as a massage oil blend.

#3

For diffuser:
3 drops rose essential oil
2 drops lavender essential oil
2 drops bergamot essential oil

Weight Loss

When you set your mind on a goal such as weight loss, these essential oils will keep you motivated and on track for your body, mind, and soul commitment to the end result.

Recommended Oils

Bergamot, clove, lavender, peppermint, sandalwood

Sample Recipes for Weight Loss

#1

1 oz. carrier oil
2 drops peppermint essential oil
3 drops clove essential oil
1 drop bergamot essential oil
Use as a massage oil blend.

#2

1 oz. carrier oil
2 drops bergamot essential oil
1 drop clove essential oil
2 drops peppermint essential oil
1 drop sandalwood essential oil
Use as a massage oil blend.

#3

For diffuser:
1 drop peppermint essential oil
2 drops bergamot essential oil
2 drop clove essential oil
1 drop sandalwood essential oil

You now have the tools to assist your body and emotions with healing. Essential oils are the first friends I seek when I need help with just about any mental or emotional challenge. You'll never know what miracles they can work until you try them.

thirty

Using Essential Oils for Spirituality and Ritual

Because essential oils have a long and rich history woven through many ages and cultures, a certain mystique has developed around them. Deep within the sacred spaces of high priests and priestesses, essential oils have achieved a lofty position of reverence and sanctity.

In the Catholic Church the holy chrism is a sacred oil mixed with olive oil and balsam essential oil. It is used for baptism, confirmation, consecration of a priest, last rights, and other high-level consecrations. Only the Bishop is allowed to make the holy chrism for the diocese.

The Balm of Gilead is mentioned in the Bible as a sacred oil for religious ceremonies. It was also composed of olive oil mixed with balsam oil. Incisions in the bark of the balsam tree yielded three to four drops per day, hence the oil was worth its weight in silver, the main measure of wealth at that time.

In Ancient Egypt, men and women about to be married anointed each other with a sacred oil that was mixed only by the high priest. It contained frankincense and myrrh, significant of cleansing and purifying.

In the recipe from the Old Testament that was allegedly given directly to Moses, the list includes galbanum and pure frankincense, in equal amounts.

Ancient Vedic rituals called for the anointing of government officials. Wise Indian Buddhists adopted and expanded the practice to include birth, initiations, marriage, deaths, ritual instruments, and new buildings.

What a splendid use of essential oils! We can take up the practice and use these glorious oils to signify the various passages of our lives and the lives of others. Think how much richer life might become. Below is an example of a ritual you can create using essential oils.

Create a Ritual to Celebrate Your Life

By this time reading the book, you should have a working knowledge of twenty different essential oils and their physical properties. Now we can begin to apply them to spiritual and magical purposes. To add depth and meaning to your life, you might consider creating a ritual for the different chapters in your life and those of your family.

In the beginning, consider the simple ones: birthdays, engagements, marriages, anniversaries, and new baby. You can commemorate other events like graduations, first jobs, housewarmings, promotions, project completion, reaching a goal, achievements, awards, citations, retirement, and other life milestones.

To create a ritual:

1. Select the essential oil or oils with the properties or qualities you want to use to commemorate the occasion.

2. Write up a special tribute to the person and invite others to speak or contribute.

3. Anoint the person, place, or thing with the essential oil (diluted of course) you have chosen to mark the occasion. Speak about the properties of the essential oil and how those qualities bring something special to the occasion and to the person.

4. Formalize the event with songs or prayers or anything you create to make it special, memorial, and meaningful for the person being celebrated.

5. Make a certificate for the person celebrated to commemorate the day.

Always let your imagination run free and have fun thinking up your own rituals and commemorations using essential oils. Especially when using and sharing the essential oil(s) you like most.

Sample Ritual (10th Anniversary)

We are gathered here today to celebrate ten years of your marriage to each other. Ten years is both a long and a short time when it comes to love and commitment. We honor you both for your patience, your kindness, your willingness to forgive, and work together to create a better world and a loving family. It has been 120 months, 521 weeks, 3,652 days, 87,729 hours, and 5,259,487 minutes since you pledged your lives to each other in marriage.

We anoint you both with (diluted) rosemary essential oil to represent protection, continued love, the warding off of any evil that might try to penetrate your bond, and as an agent to keep you youthful and in the spirit of the day you first said your vows.

We also anoint you with (diluted) rose so that you may continue to attract love and keep each other close. Rose signifies the deepest feelings of love and compassion, keeping always the personal connection you have to each other and that it may last and endure through all the days and nights of your life together.

The commemorative certificate might read:

On this date: _____

We honor (name and name)

On the Occasion of their Tenth Anniversary—120 months, 521 weeks, 3,652 days, 87,729 hours, and 5,259,487 minutes—of loving one another and sharing that love with the world.

Long may they live, thrive, and prosper

Add a lined area for the signatures of all people who celebrated them on this day.

Celebrating a Birthday

You can easily celebrate someone's birthday by selecting an essential oil for them that represents their astrological sign. In the list below you can find the sign by birthdate. Under the date and sign are essential oils listed that are compatible with that sign. The essential oils suggested compliment the person of that zodiac sign and help them enhance their astrological characteristics and traits. Personalize their gift with an astrological reading you obtain for them and a lovely diffuser or nebulizer so they can be surrounded by scents that complement their sign. Below are some suggestions for a sign-specific birthday treat.

Essential Oils for Aries: March 21–April 19
Pine, frankincense, lemon, rosemary, peppermint, rose, Roman chamomile, lavender, clove

Essential Oils for Taurus: April 20–May 20
Black pepper, rosemary, lemon, eucalyptus, Roman chamomile, patchouli, ylang-ylang

Essential Oils for Gemini: May 21–June 20
Lavender, thyme, eucalyptus bergamot, geranium, Roman chamomile

Essential Oils for Cancer: June 21–July 22
Peppermint, bergamot, Roman chamomile, rosemary, lavender

Essential Oils for Leo: July 23–August 22
Lemon, rosemary, rose, Melissa, orange

Essential Oils for Virgo: August 23–September 22
Ylang-ylang, Roman chamomile, Melissa, lemon, thyme

Essential Oils for Libra: September 23–October 22
Rose, geranium, bergamot, lavender, frankincense, clary sage

Essential Oils for Scorpio: October 23–November 21
Patchouli, ylang-ylang, sandalwood, clary sage, lavender, geranium

Essential Oils for Sagittarius: November 22–December 21
Tea tree, eucalyptus, geranium, rosemary, lavender, frankincense

Essential Oils for Capricorn: December 22–January 19
Eucalyptus, tea tree, lavender, rosemary, lemon, patchouli, sandalwood, bergamot, Melissa

Essential Oils for Aquarius: January 20–February 18
Lemon, peppermint, rose, Roman chamomile, geranium, eucalyptus

Essential Oils for Pisces: February 19–March 20
Rosemary, peppermint, bergamot, lavender, sandalwood, patchouli, rose, frankincense

Create an Intention, Meditation, or Affirmation

In the next section you'll learn about many different ways essential oils can be applied for spiritual use. If one or two of the suggestions speak to you or are exactly what you feel you need to hear, perhaps you can set the suggestion as an intention for your yoga practice or meditation. Jot down the suggestion and write it into a complete sentence that becomes an affirmation of what you want to learn or incorporate into your life.

For example: Melissa suggests that you diffuse that essential oil if you want to find an appreciation of past-life lessons and incorporate them into your life so you can move forward with wisdom. The affirmation for that desire would read something like: *In a spirit of gratitude, I celebrate the renewed wisdom in my life by seeing clearly how my past-life experiences have contributed to making me the person I am today.*

Turn what you wish for into a positive statement that you already have obtained what you seek. Meditate on this statement in the presence of the essential oil suggested and see how your heart opens and your soul experience deepens. You can repeat the same process for all the ideas and suggestions that touch you as relevant to your growth and development.

Metaphysical Properties of the Twenty Essential Oils

If you want to incorporate essential oils in your practices, readings, ceremonies, and everyday spiritual practices, you might find this section helpful. I have compiled a list of the essential oils mentioned in this book and their magical and spiritual backgrounds. Many of these ideas have been handed down through generations over centuries. I believe that when you set your intention for something and use a specific essential oil to enhance that intention, you open your world to the realm of possibility and fulfillment. Nothing can be considered silly if it is useful and effective. Try some of these out yourself. See what happens.

You can use these oils in your meditation practice, during your yoga session, or you can place a few drops on a cotton ball and carry it with you to inspire you when you have something to accomplish. Many of the essential oils are for attracting love, some are for prosperity and abundance, and some are for healing various human emotions. There are suggestions for the use of each oil listed below. Use them on a piece of cloth you carry with you, in a special magical bag with your oil-doused cloth, crystals, or talismans. Decide what you want to accomplish and choose the essential oil with the properties to attract that action. Add a crystal or stone imbued with similar attracting qualities or an icon that represents completed success. You will develop even more creative ways to incorporate these aromas into your spiritual life for healing and the magnification of your spirit.

Bergamot (Citrus bergamia) Essential Oil

- Used to elevate the spirit, clarify the mind, and assist with confidence-building and inner strength. Bergamot essential oil helps to overcome disempowerment, victim consciousness, despondency, and helps to connect to one's higher self, highest calling, and inner purpose.
- Place several drops of bergamot essential oil on a one-inch cloth square and slip into your wallet or purse to build confidence.
- A few drops of bergamot essential oil can be used in rituals to attract success and casting spells.

- Add bergamot essential oil to a diffuser to help you stay connected to your life's purpose and meaning.

- Place one to two drops of bergamot essential oil on a one-inch piece of cloth to protect yourself from being a victim or attracting people who want to use you.

- *Affirmative Statement: I experience clarity of thought which gives me the power to realize that I am equal to the brightest lights, sharpest minds, and boldest persons on this planet.*

Clary Sage (Salvia sclarea) Essential Oil

- Enhances dreaming; is protective, calming, and balancing; brings in wisdom of the sages; and lifts melancholy, paranoia, and stress.

- Sprinkle drops of clary sage essential oil around the table you lay out your tarot cards, runes, bones, or stones.

- Rub two drops of clary sage essential oil in your hands and inhale its fragrance to elicit inner wisdom.

- For a personal aura cleanse, mix twenty-five drops of clary sage essential oil with one half teaspoon of vodka in a 50-ml mist bottle filled with spring water. Spritz, don't drink. (Vodka or witch hazel helps disperse the oil and keeps it mixed with the water.)

- Mix two drops of clary sage essential oil with one cup of warm water to make an excellent clearing and enhancing wash for scrying mirrors and scrying stones.

- Diffuse clary sage essential oil or anoint the third eye during metaphysical activities to enhance your visioning abilities and the reading.

- A drop or two of clary sage essential oil placed on a cloth or tissue under your pillow can enhance any dream work and aid in the recall of dreams, especially for divination purposes.

- Clary sage essential oil enhances the ability to dream vividly. Mix five drops of clary sage essential oil with five drops of thyme essential oil and diffuse before bedtime.

- To connect with the universal energies, mix one drop of clary sage essential oil with one drop of bergamot essential oil. Place on a cotton ball and inhale deeply.

- *Affirmative Statement: My heart, soul, and dreams lift me into realms of wisdom where balance and joy reign supreme and I am at one with and connected to the ease of living in joy.*

Clove Bud (Syzygium aromaticum) Essential Oil

- Clove bud is good for protection, exorcism, and love.

- Place two drops of clove bud essential oil on a one-inch piece of cloth which is on your body to attract the opposite sex.

- Place two drops of clove bud essential oil on a sachet of lavender to comfort the bereaved and those suffering from grief or loss.

- Wear a few drops of clove bud essential oil in a diffuser necklace to protect against negative forces and to purify the space around you.

- Diffuse four drops of clove bud essential oil to tonify the air and attract riches.

- Add one drop of clove bud essential oil to the largest bill in your wallet to attract money.

- Diffuse two drops of clove bud essential oil and one drop of bergamot to halt gossipers.

- *Affirmative Statement: I am protected by the invisible cloak of eternal love and universal light that surrounds me all the days and nights of my life.*

Eucalyptus (Eucalyptus globulus. E radiata) Essential Oil

- Eucalyptus essential oil clears the air and is used for healing physical and emotional issues that are blocked or stuck. It is used for protection, good health, and warding off intruders.

- Place a few drops of eucalyptus essential oil on a small piece of cloth and place beneath your pillow to ward off colds or low resistance.

- Place a few drops of eucalyptus essential oil on a one-inch cloth square and sniff it during times of emotional upset or in the presence of emotional triggers.

- Diffuse eucalyptus essential oil during meditation when you want to break through nagging issues.

- Diffuse eucalyptus essential oil at the new year or on your birthday when you want to make positive changes in your life and anoint the upcoming year.

- Place a few drops of eucalyptus essential oil on a talisman and carry it as protection against unwanted interlopers.

- *Affirmative Statement: I breathe in fresh energy that permeates my physical and emotional body and opens* up the flowing, healing channels of perfect health, safety, and balance.

Frankincense (Boswellia carteri) Essential Oil

- Frankincense essential oil promotes acceptance, emotional balance, and stability; offers protection, fortitude, courage, and resolution; increases introspection, spiritual awareness, and inspiration; and aids in meditative practices and prayer work.

- Frankincense essential oil can be used as an anointing oil for ceremonies, rituals, and rites of passage.

- Diffuse for meditation to access awareness and inspiration.

- Honor ancestors by placing a drop of frankincense beneath their picture or near a keepsake.

- Amulets coated with frankincense can bring protection and strength to the wearer.

- *Affirmative Statement: I am supported, loved, stable, and secure, and in that awareness I rise to inspire and connect with my inner meaning and purpose, and thereby serve the world.*

Lavender (Lavandula angustifolia) Essential Oil

- In occult and magical practice, lavender essential oil is used to attract love, incite prophetic dreams, open the third eye, and encourage the appearance of spirits. Lavender has historically been used as a gift offering to various deities, and as a form of incense for cleansing and consecration.

- For wishes to come true, place drops of lavender essential oil on your pillow as you bring the wish to mind. (First test the pillow fabric for oil staining.)
- Infuse clothing with lavender essential oil to attract love.
- Drop lavender essential oil on stationery for writing enticing love notes.
- Wear lavender essential oil on clothing to promote long life.
- *Affirmative Statement: I am lifted into higher realms where I can readily access my gifts and connect to the others who have walked my path and who will guide me along my journey.*

Lemon (Citrus x limon) Essential Oil

- Lemon represents longevity, purification, love, and friendship.
- Use one drop of lemon essential oil on a one-inch piece of cloth and place beneath your visitor's chair and the friendship will be made permanent.
- Wash used amulets, magical objects, and other second-hand jewelry in lemon essential oil and water to remove any negative vibrations.
- Use a drop or two of lemon essential oil on stationery and cards to enhance friendship.
- After a break-up or separation, use a lemon essential oil spray to purify the space and create room for new love.

- *Affirmative Statement: I now connect to others in a spirit of friendship, love, mutual appreciation, and support as we move through our long lives as beings dedicated to a purpose of sharing.*

Melissa (Melissa officinalis) Essential Oil

- Melissa attracts gentleness, peace, forgiveness, love, success, healing, and brings in the energy of the spirit.
- Diffuse Melissa essential oil for appreciation of past-life lessons and for incorporating them into your life today and moving forward with wisdom.
- To receive understanding and support, diffuse or inhale Melissa essential oil (over steam or rub into your palms, diluted and inhaled) or dab a few drops on a one-inch piece of cloth and put under your pillow.
- Before your meditation, place two drops of Melissa essential oil onto a cotton ball, inhale, and you can expect some help with a spiritual awakening or breakthrough.
- A few drops of diluted Melissa essential oil sprinkled on the body brings happiness.
- *Affirmative Statement: In a spirit of gratitude, I celebrate the renewed wisdom in my life by seeing clearly how my past-life experiences have contributed to making me the person I am today.*

Orange (Citrus sinensis) Essential Oil

- Orange promotes love, divination, luck, and money.
- A few drops of orange essential oil placed on the flowers of a wedding bouquet leads to wedded bliss.

- The Chinese believe orange essential oil brings good luck and fortune. Drops of the oil on money or coins bring prosperity.

- Diffused orange essential oil will draw abundance to the home.

- Place a few drops of orange essential oil above your doorway to welcome luck and money.

- *Affirmative Statement: Prosperity surrounds me and I feel abundant, fortunate, and blessed with love and everything I need for a happy life.*

Patchouli (Pogostemon cablin) Essential Oil

- Patchouli essential oil has a spicy, deep earthy scent and is frequently used because of its connection to the rich earth. Civilizations have counted on it to bring prosperity and abundance to homes and families. The oil is used in ceremonies and prayers for those who need financial or other types of blessings in their lives.

- One drop of patchouli essential oil is often combined with one drop of sandalwood or rose essential oil to attract love. Use on a one-inch piece of cloth and carry with you or place beneath your pillow at night.

- Moisten a cotton ball with one to two drops of patchouli essential oil. Close your eyes and visualize the cash rolling in as you inhale to activate your attraction of money.

- Diffuse a few drops of patchouli essential oil to attract a partner and to heighten lust.

- Diffused patchouli essential oil seems to lower sexual inhibitions in women, and lowers anxiety in men, thus improving sexual enjoyment for both sexes.

- Anoint an icon representing children with patchouli essential oil, place it in a location where you can see it every day, and children will manifest.

- *Affirmative Statement: Tapping into the wisdom of the past, I use this connection to know that I am blessed, one with the earth and ready to receive of all her generous and abundant gifts.*

Peppermint (Mentha x piperita) Essential Oil

- Peppermint essential oil brings about purification, love, sleep, healing, and psychic powers.

- A drop of diluted peppermint essential oil worn on the wrist can ward off negative thoughts and energy.

- Sniffed or inhaled, peppermint essential oil encourages a magical dream-filled sleep.

- Drops of peppermint essential oil on a cloth placed beneath the pillow bring on dreams of the future.

- Drops of peppermint essential oil diluted and rubbed lightly on furniture wards off evil. (Be sure to pre-test surfaces first).

- Enhance your psychic powers by diffusing a few drops of peppermint essential oil.

- Pliny the Elder, Roman author and naturalist, wrote, "peppermint excites love," so peppermint essential oil can be added to a love potion.

- Place two drops of peppermint essential oil on a small one-inch cloth and place in the wallet for prosperity.
- *Affirmative Statement: Enthusiastically I claim perfection in body, mind, and spirit for myself and gratefully accept the natural healing that I am entitled to receive as member of the human race.*

Pine (Pinus sylvestris) Essential Oil

- Pine essential oil contains the powers of fertility, healing, and protection.
- Drops of pine essential oil on a one-inch piece of cloth worn by the person can promote fertility.
- Sprinkle pine essential oil on a branch and hang above the front door for protection and to keep joy within the walls.
- To keep sickness away, hang a pine cone dotted with drops of pine essential oil above the bed to ward off germs.
- Use pine essential oil for money attraction. Place a few drops on a $5 bill and keep in your wallet.
- To ward off negative or evil spirits, dilute pine essential oil with water in a spray bottle and spray around the perimeter of your house.
- *Affirmative Statement: I have the ability to create anything I want to create because I am loved, protected, and cherished as a vibrant child of this unlimited universe.*

Rose (Rosa x damascena) Essential Oil

- Rose essential oil is used to promote healing, love, luxury, contentment, protection, happiness, and unconditional love. Rose essential oil unites the physical with the spiritual.

- It is said that when you inhale rose essential oil, you inhale the love and kisses of angels.
- To attract and keep love, apply a few drops of rose essential oil to note paper for sending love letters.
- For personal contentment, apply a few drops of rose essential oil onto a one-inch piece of cloth and place beneath your pillow.
- Place two drops of diluted rose essential oil on your palms, rub together, and inhale for protection, healing, and self-confidence.
- Rose essential oil diffused in a magical setting will summon your deepest feelings.
- *Affirmative Statement: At the deepest place where my heart and soul reside, I know the true meaning of love and happiness and it fills me with joy every day of my life.*

Roman Chamomile (Chamaemelum nobile) Essential Oil

- Roman chamomile essential oil brings love, money, purification, and sleep.
- Sprinkled around a property, it is believed to remove curses.
- Patted above a doorway, it can provide protection and bring happiness to the inhabitants.
- A few drops on a one-inch cloth placed under a pillow brings a peaceful and calm night's sleep.

- Two drops on a one-inch cloth sniffed gently relieves tension and worry.

- *Affirmative Statement: I rest in absolute assurance that I am supplied with everything I need to be a loved, prosperous, abundant, and productive person.*

Rose Geranium (Pelargonium graveolens) Essential Oil

- Rose geranium is good for fertility, health, love, and protection.

- Diffuse three to four drops of rose geranium essential oil to release negative memories, ease nervous tension, balance emotions, lift your spirits, and to summon peace, well-being, and optimism.

- Use rose geranium essential oil to inspire natural beauty, to tonify the mind, and to mobilize hidden creative and emotional reserves. Inhale, diffuse, or carry drops with you on a small piece of cloth.

- Diffused rose geranium essential oil helps crystalize earthly and spiritual identities.

- Use drops of rose geranium essential oil in spells and rituals for stirring up spirit and passion.

- Place two drops of rose geranium essential oil on a one-inch piece of cloth and place under your pillow along with a photo of your beloved. This will create a love spell for the relationship.

- Make a sachet and add three drops of rose geranium essential oil for guardianship. Place sachets in areas of the house where you need protection.

- Rub a few drops of rose geranium essential oil above doorways and windows to ward off intruders. (Test the surface before anointing in case of staining.)
- *Affirmative Statement: Optimism fills me, easing my pain and bringing me to a state of gratitude for everything in my past and present with all the blessings, health, and well-being that I enjoy every day.*

Rosemary (Rosmarinus officinalis) Essential Oil

- Rosemary is used to bring protection, love, lust, purification, healing, and sleep; enhance mental powers; exorcise evil spirits; and as an agent for youth.
- Use a few drops of rosemary essential oil in hotel rooms to increase safety and help your body adapt to a strange location.
- A drop of rosemary essential oil on a cloth under your pillow will help chase nightmares away.
- If you want an answer to a question, burn a drop of rosemary essential oil on a charcoal brick, gently inhale a bit of the smoke, and the answer will come to you.
- Diffuse a few drops of rosemary essential oil to increase mental clarity and raise feelings of safety and protection.
- Keep a cotton ball with two drops of rosemary essential oil handy when you are concentrating and need to break away. Sniff every hour for mental refreshment and clarity.
- *Affirmative Statement: Purified and youthful in my soul, mind, and body, I am surrounded by positive ele-*

ments that protect me from danger and allow me to rest and heal from the pressures that can come from a dedicated and busy life.

Sandalwood (Santalum album) Essential Oil

- Sandalwood is good for protection, full moon rituals, healing, exorcism, past lives, and to encourage wishes to come true.
- Sandalwood essential oil awakens sensuality and invokes calm and deep relaxation. It opens the cellular memory of past-life experiences.
- Diffuse a few drops with lavender essential oil to conjure spirits.
- Diffuse or mix a few drops with frankincense essential oil for full moon rituals and anointing.
- Write your wish on a three-inch piece of cloth and drop sandalwood essential oil on it. Place under your pillow and visualize it coming true.
- Place a few drops of diluted sandalwood essential oil on a cotton ball and inhale to help recall past-life experiences.
- Sandalwood essential oil can be used in bereavement ceremonies to help with the crossing-over process and to ease the sense of loss for the mourners.
- Sandalwood essential oil is also used in many forms of initiation rites to open the disciple's mind to receive consecration.
- *Affirmative Statement: Connecting to lunar energy, I activate my inner power and know that whatever path*

I take, whatever my next move is, I will be successful, blessed, and protected as my desires are fulfilled.

Tea Tree (Melaleuca alternifolia) Essential Oil

- In occult and magical practice, tea tree essential oil is used to enhance strength; to cleanse, protect, and purify; and to open and focus the channels of the mind for more clarity. It is also used for opening the upper chakras.
- Place a drop of tea tree essential oil on a one-inch piece of cloth to carry with you in situations where you could use some extra strength and courage.
- Inhale two drops of tea tree essential oil rubbed on the palms of your hands to open upper chakras and to increase mental clarity.
- Cleanse away all negative energies by adding a drop of tea tree essential oil to a cotton ball and inhaling three times.
- *Affirmative Statement. My mind is enlivened, my spirits are elevated, and I am cleansed of all negative energies as I exercise strength in everything I think and do.*

Thyme (Thymus vulgaris) Essential Oil

- Thyme is excellent for attracting good health, instilling courage, removing past darkness, and connecting with the fourth dimension.
- Drops of thyme essential oil on a one-inch piece of cloth can attract good health.

- Use drops of thyme essential oil on a piece of one-inch cloth for healing spells. Or diffuse thyme during the spell.

- A few drops of thyme essential oil placed on a cloth beneath a pillow bring restful sleep without nightmares.

- A magical, cleansing bath of properly dispersed thyme essential oil drops removes past sorrows and ills.

- Drops of thyme essential oil worn on clothing allow the wearer to see faeries.

- A drop of thyme essential oil on clothing will give the wearer extra courage.

- Sniffed, thyme essential oil will bring courage and energy to any situation. Use a drop or two on a cotton ball and sniff gently.

- Diffused thyme essential oil will purify your space.

- *Affirmative Statement: I am empowered to successfully face anything that crosses my path with courage and illumination, because I connect to any realm I choose for wisdom and assistance.*

Ylang-Ylang (Cananga odorata) Essential Oil

- Ylang-ylang is wonderful for enhancing calm and is uplifting, enthusiastic, and joyful.

- Use a few drops of ylang-ylang essential oil for love spells and potions.

- Add a few drops of ylang-ylang essential oil to a piece of cloth and place under your pillow to attract a love interest.

- Add a few drops of ylang-ylang essential oil to a piece of cloth and place under your pillow to reduce fear or apprehension
- *Affirmative Statement: In an elegant state of peace, I experience the uplifting serenity that joy brings, and I am filled with enthusiasm and appreciation for all the facets of my life.*

———————

In our busy lives we often forget to include essential oils in our spiritual practices or use them in the process of healing our souls. As we deal with the chapters of our lives and face the obstacles that grow our character and turn us into everyday heroes, let us bring essential oils into the fold and count on their natural benefits to aid us along our path. They bring us healing, rejuvenation, and transformation in the form of the countless blessings they can bestow if we invite them in to participate with us on our expedition.

final thoughts

Congratulations on making the journey through the beginner's course for essential oils. You will find that there are many more essential oils available in this abundant natural world of ours than the ones we covered in this book. The count is well over 400[14] in circulation today. You have acres of diamonds ahead of you to explore.

Essential oils do more than just smell good. They heal us and our planet on several levels. Many rural civilizations in third-world countries are farming plants and trees to produce

---

14. Robert Tisserand and Rodney Young, *Essential Oils Safety second edition* (United Kingdom: Churchill Livingstone Elsevier, 2014), xiii.

essential oils and are turning their economies around using sustainable practices without pesticides.

Researchers continue to experiment with essential oils and test the results of healing claims and chemical properties. Progress is being made in scientific laboratories around the world as researchers delve deeper into the chemical properties, qualities, and benefits that essential oils provide to the human body. The future for essential oils and their application to human betterment is wide open, and we are sure to learn more in the coming years from the diligent work of researchers and essential oil experts around the globe.

Essential oils play a big part in holistic treatment and integrated medicine practices. Western medicine and alternative healing practices are beginning to overlap and share their discoveries and successes. What seemed to be on the fringe decades ago is now becoming mainstream. And it's only going to get better from here.

In many cultures we are already using ancient knowledge with modern technology to help ourselves and our planet. It's a very exciting time to be alive.

Now that you have acquired a basic understanding of essential oils and their uses, the next time you need a remedy you'll have even more options at your disposal that can best serve your needs. Having more choices gives you brand-new horizons to explore. Welcome to your new world of natural oils and the abundant future they have in store for you.

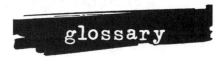

glossary

Analgesic: Pain relieving
Anti-allergenic: Reduces symptoms of allergies
Antibacterial: Fights bacterial growth
Antiblastic: Prevents parasite growth
Anti-cancerous: Inhibits growth of cancer cells
Anticonvulsant: Helps control convulsions
Antidepressant: Helps to counteract depression and lifts the mood
Antifungal: Prevents fungi growth
Anti-inflammatory: Reduces inflammation
Antimicrobial: Reduces or resists microbes
Antiphlogistic: Counteracts inflammation

Antipyretic: Reduces fever

Antirheumatic: Helps to combat rheumatism

Anti-seborrheic: Fights a skin condition that causes scaly patches and red skin, mainly on the scalp

Antiseptic: Helps control infection

Antispasmodic: Helps to control spasms

Antitumoral: Inhibits the development of tumors

Antitussive: Relieves coughing

Antiviral: Counteracts the effects of viruses

Aperitif: Stimulates the appetite

Aphrodisiac: Increases sexual desire and sexual functioning

Aromatic: Having a pleasant and distinctive smell

Astringent: Causes skin tissue to contract; good for toning skin

Autoimmune disease: A disease in which the body's immune system attacks healthy cells

Bactericide: Destroys bacteria

Cardiotonic: Exerting a favorable, so-called tonic effect on the action of the heart

Carminative: Settles the digestive system and relieves flatulence

Cephalic: Stimulating and clearing the mind

Cholagogue: Promotes the secretion of bile into the duodenum

Cicatrisant: Promotes healing by scar tissue formation

Cordial: A heart tonic

Cytophylactic: Increases the leukocyte activity to defend the body against infection

Deodorant: Works against and masks body odor

Depurative: Helps to detoxify and to combat impurities in the blood and body

Detoxifier: Combats impurities in the blood and body

Diaphoretic: Helps to promote perspiration

Digestive: Helps digestion

Disinfectant: Causes the destruction of bacteria

Diuretic: Helps increase the production of urine

Emmenagogue: Promotes and stimulates menstrual flow

Emollient: Softening and soothing to the skin

Euphoric: Feeling intense excitement and happiness

Expectorant: Helps to expel mucus from the lungs

Febrifuge: Helps to combat fever

Fungicidal: Inhibiting the growth of fungi

Fungicide: Destroys fungal infections

Haemostatic: Retarding or stopping bleeding

Hemostatic: Arresting hemorrhage, styptic

Hepatic: A tonic for the liver

Hypotensive: Lowers blood pressure

Immune stimulant: Induces activation or increases activity of any of the components of the immune system

Laxative: Helps with bowel movements

Lymphatic stimulant: Promotes lymph flow, which in turn removes waste products

Memory enhancer: Promotes better memory recall

Metabolic stimulant: Boosts the rate at which body processes function

Nervine: Strengthens and tones the nerves and nervous system

Parasiticide: Kills parasites (especially those other than bacteria or fungi)

Rubefacient: Causes redness of the skin by stimulating blood circulation

Relaxant: Promotes relaxation or reduces tension

Restorative: Restores health, strength, or a feeling of well-being

Reviving: Gives new strength or energy

Sedative: Provides a soothing and calming effect

Skin tonic: Tones, stimulates, or freshens the skin

Stimulant: Provides an invigorating action on the body and circulation

Stomach tonic: Helps digestion and improves appetite

Stomachic: Promotes the appetite or assists digestion

Styptic: Capable of stopping bleeding when applied to a wound

Sudorific: Induces sweating

Tonic: Gives a feeling of vigor or well-being; invigorating

Uterine: Relating to the uterus or womb

Uterine agent: Induces contraction or greater tonicity of the uterus

Vasodilator: Causes vasodilatation, the dilatation of blood vessels

Vermifuge: Expels intestinal worms

Vulnerary: Helps to heal wounds and sores and helps to prevent tissue degeneration

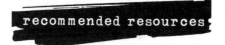
recommended resources

General

American Botanical Council: Herbal medicine information that includes an herb library and clinical guide to herbs. http://abc.herbalgram.org/.

AromaWeb: A directory of aromatherapy information, tips, recipes, sources, including a regional aromatherapy business directory and school. https://www.aromaweb.com/.

HerbMed: Interactive electronic herb database (some information is free, but full access requires a fee). http://www.herbmed.org/.

National Association for Holistic Aromatherapy (NAHA): Questions answered about the medicinal use of aromatic

plants and the holistic practice of aromatherapy. https://
naha.org/.

Pub Med Central. Source for research and papers on the
science of essential oils. https://www.ncbi.nlm.nih.gov/
pmc/?term=Essential+oils.

Overall Safety

https://www.naha.org/explore-aromatherapy/safety

Animal Safety

https://naha.org/assets/uploads/Animal_Aromatherapy
_Safety_NAHA.pdf

Pregnancy Safety

https://naha.org/explore-aromatherapy/safety Scroll to
pregnancy guidelines.

Finding a Certified Aromatherapist

https://naha.org/find-an-aromatherapist

source material

Book Sources

Cunningham, Scott. *Cunningham's Encyclopedia of Magical Herbs*. Woodbury, MN: Llewellyn Worldwide, 2013.

Essential Oils Natural Remedies. New York, NY: Fall River Press, Althea Press, 2015.

Garland, Sarah. *The Complete Book of Herbs and Spices*. London, France: Lincoln Ltd., 2004.

Harris, Ben Charles. *The Complete Herbal*. New York: Larchmont Books, 1972.

Lawless, Julia. *The Complete Illustrated Guide to Aromatherapy*. New York, NY: Barnes & Noble Books, 2003.

Schnaubelt, Kurt. *The Healing Intelligence of Essential Oils.* Rochester, VT: Healing Arts Press, 2011.

Tisserand, Robert, Rodney Young. *Essential Oil Safety: A Guide for Health Care Professionals.* London, UK: Churchill Livingstone, 2002.

Worwood, Valerie Ann. *The Complete Book of Essential Oils and Aromatherapy.* Novato, CA: New World Library, 1991.

Young, Kac. *The Healing Art of Essential Oils.* Woodbury, MN: Llewellyn Publications, 2017.

Tisserand, Robert, Rodney Young. *Essential Oil Safety.* London, Churchill Livingstone, Elsevier, 2014.

Web Sources

Avicenna. *The Canon of Medicine (work by Avicenna). Encyclopædia Britannica. 2008. Archived from the original on 28 May 2008. Retrieved 2008-06-11.* May 28. Accessed February 4, 2019.

Chakrabordy, HC Chandola and Arunangschu. 2009. *Fibromyalgia and Myofascial Pain Syndrome-A Dilemma.* October 5. Accessed December 23, 2018. https://www.ncbi.nlm.nih.gov/pmc/articles/PMC2900090/#CIT21

n.d. *https://mymerrymessylife.com/12-essential-oils-of-ancient-scripture-webinar-notes-and-video.*

n.d. *Chamomille, herbs-info.com, http://www.herbs-info.com/chamomile.html* accessed October 2, 2015.

Howell, Jeremy. 2010. *BBC World News.* February 9. Accessed December 15, 2018. http://news.bbc.co.uk/2/hi/middle_east/8505251.stm.

n.d. *Johns Hopkins Packs Vs Warm Compresses for Pain.* Accessed Jan 22, 2019. https://www.hopkinsmedicine.org/healthlibrary/conditions/orthopaedic_disorders/ice_packs_vs_warm_compresses_for_pain_85,p00918.

Klimczak, Natalia. 2017. *The Forgotten Cleopatra: Searching for Cleopatra the Alchemist and Her Golden Secret.* February 21. Accessed February 5, 2019. https://www.ancient-origins.net/history-famous-people/forgotten-cleopatra-searching-cleopatra-alchemist-and-her-golden-secret-007585.

Linden., Stanton J. 2003. "The Alchemy Reader: From Hermes Trismegistus to Isaac Newton. Cambridge University Press. 2003. p.44." In *The Alchemy Reader: From Hermes Trismegistus to Isaac Newton,* by Stanton J. Linden, 44. Cambridge: Cambridge University Press.

Soloway, Rose Ann Gould. 2010. *National Capital Poison Center.* Accessed January 15, 2019. https://www.poison.org/articles/2010-dec/tea-tree-oil.

Woodbine, Robert. n.d. *Essential Oils From Past to Present.* Accessed February 15, 2019. https://www.goread.com/buzz/rob-thomas-2/article/essential-oils-from-the-past-to-the-present/.

n.d. *World Wide Science.org.* Accessed February 2, 2019. https://worldwidescience.org/topicpages/p/plant+essential+oil.html.

index

A

Acne, 59–61, 64, 72, 73, 85, 101, 112, 127, 150, 168, 178–180, 186, 250

Addiction, 251

Adults, 9, 36, 37, 126, 137, 224, 244, 256

Aging skin, 60, 251, 253

Allergens, 59, 155, 329

Analgesic, 20, 58–60, 72, 85, 119, 137, 155, 168, 329

Anaphylactic, 35, 39, 40

Anger, 29, 119, 121, 150, 151, 161, 191, 193, 263, 288

Antiaging, 58, 59, 61, 62, 64, 65, 175

S

To Write to the Author

If you wish to contact the author or would like more information about this book, please write to the author in care of Llewellyn Worldwide, and we will forward your request. Both the author and publisher appreciate hearing from you and learning of your enjoyment of this book and how it has helped you. Llewellyn Worldwide cannot guarantee that every letter written to the author can be answered, but all will be forwarded. Please write to:

Kac Young, PhD
℅ Llewellyn Worldwide
2143 Wooddale Drive
Woodbury, MN 55125.2989

Please enclose a self-addressed stamped envelope for reply, or $1.00 to cover costs. If outside the U.S.A., enclose an international postal reply coupon.